JUST BREATHE

Meditation made simple

pil

Publications International, Ltd.

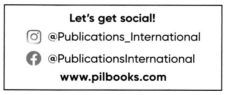

Let's get social!
@Publications_International
@PublicationsInternational
www.pilbooks.com

TABLE OF CONTENTS

Why Meditate? 4

Just Breathe. 16

Setting the Scene 35

Meditations 54

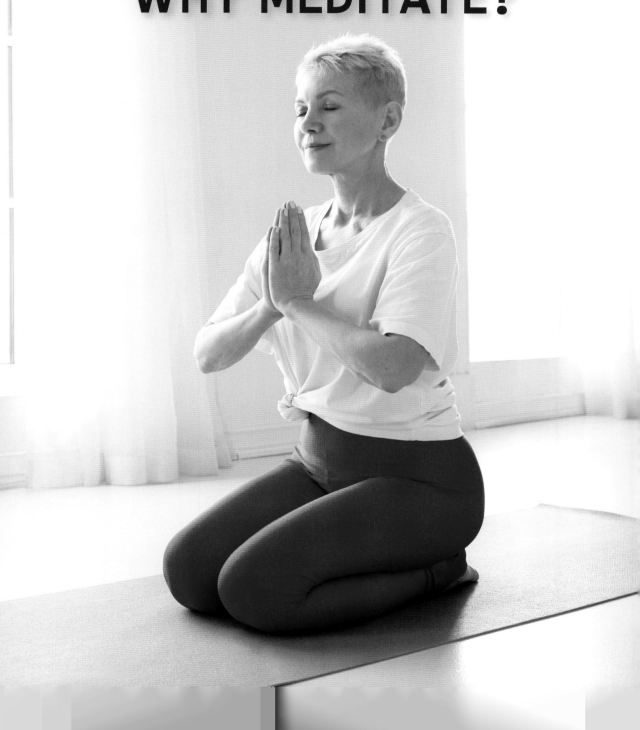

WHY MEDITATE?

WELCOME TO MEDITATION

Meditation actively trains the mind to cultivate awareness, focus, and clarity. This is primarily done through focused attention. Left to its own devices, the mind can bombard a person with an uncontrolled waterfall of thoughts. Meditation can help turn this waterfall into a steadier, more manageable stream. Like any other form of exercise, meditation comes more easily with time and practice.

Over the millennia and around the world, people have meditated with a variety of intentions and methods. For some, meditation is part of their religious practice or spiritual journey. It is disciplined devotion that brings the practitioner closer to the divine. To other people, it is entirely secular. Meditation may be done in movement or stillness, with sound or in silence, over hours or minutes.

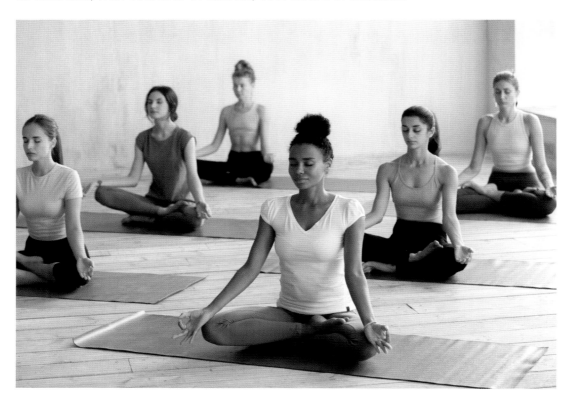

BENEFITS

A number of benefits can come from meditating. Depending on the meditation technique you use, you might see more of some benefits over others. Research so far has suggested:

- Meditation increases your ability to concentrate.
- It can improve your memory and thought processes.
- It helps preserve your brain as it ages, resulting in less gray matter loss.
- It helps with stress-related illnesses such as anxiety, depression, irritable bowel syndrome, and insomnia.
- It may help reduce the severity of menopausal symptoms, including hot flashes, muscle and joint pain, and changes in sleep and mood.

- It might reduce asthma symptoms.
- It can reduce your blood pressure.
- It can help fight the habit of rumination, or prolonged focus on negative or distressing thoughts.
- It may help reduce inflammation and pain.
- It causes changes in the areas of the brain that regulate emotion.
- It may help treat addiction by causing changes in the parts of the brain that deal with self-control.
- It can increase compassion, felt for both yourself and others.

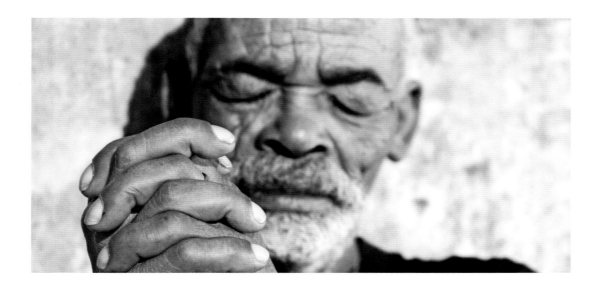

IS MEDITATION FOR ME?

Yes! Meditation can be for anyone. It might take a few tries before you find the right method for you, or some practice before it becomes a comfortable routine, but whoever you are, whatever your circumstances, you can meditate.

Meditation does not have to cost money. The only real necessity is time. Additional things—a special cushion, a yoga mat, some guided meditations—require payment, but it's entirely possible to meditate without them. In addition, meditation is accessible and adaptable. Everyone has a unique set of limitations and abilities. If one approach doesn't work for you, try another. There are so many ways to meditate and so many ways to modify those methods.

When you're looking for a place to start with meditation, consider what you need and what you want:

Need stillness?
Try a seated meditation.

Like to move?
You can walk or try Qigong or yoga.

Strapped for time?
Try a short breathing exercise.

Not a morning person?
Meditate in the afternoon or evening, and vice versa.

Can't concentrate in silence?
Have calm music playing in the background, or repeat a mantra aloud.

Uncomfortable in a position?
Modify it.

Can't enter a position at all?
Try a different one: lie down, kneel, stretch your legs out, stand.

Does a physical object help you concentrate?
Count on a string of beads or focus your eyes on a candle or image.

As you read this book, keep an eye out for information and activities that spark your interest. This can be a sign you've found a good place to begin.

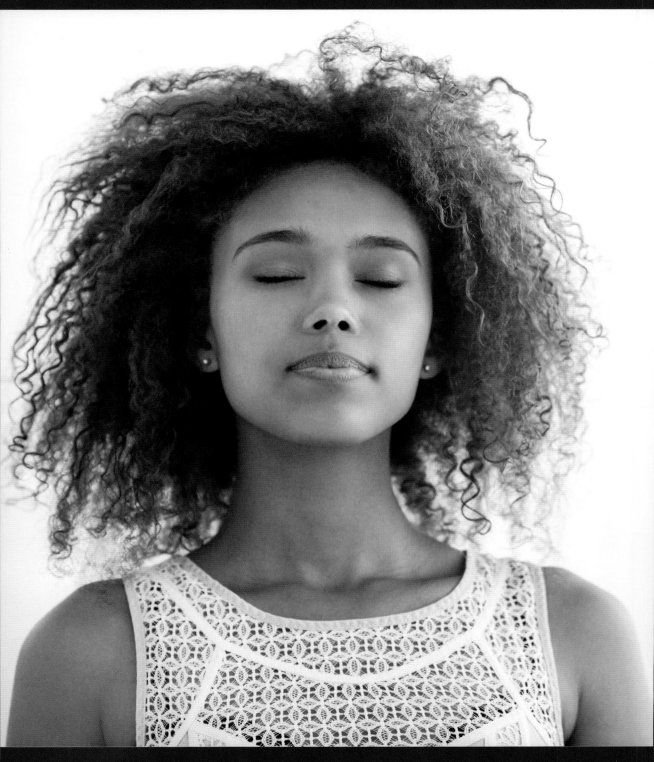

You may retire into yourself at any hour you please. Nowhere can a man find any retreat more quiet and more full of leisure than in his own soul; especially when there is that within it on which, if he but look, he is straightway quite at rest. And rest I hold to be naught else but perfect order in the soul.

—Marcus Aurelius

Stillness—

the cicada's cry

drills into the rocks.

　　　—Matsuo Basho

　　　The earth

　　　laughs in flowers.

　　　—Ralph Waldo Emerson

　　　　　experimenting

　　　　　I hung the moon on

　　　　　various branches of pine.

　　　　　　—Hokushi

BETTER HEALTH THROUGH MEDITATION

Meditation does more than bring a sense of calm, emotional balance, and well-being into your life. The benefits include better overall health—and these don't end when your meditation sessions end. In fact, some people report lifelong benefits from meditation after only six months of daily practice.

If you have a medical condition, particularly one worsened by stress, meditation may help with the attendant anxiety or pain. Scientific research suggests other conditions, such as tension headaches, chronic pain, sleep problems, asthma, depression, high blood pressure, and irritable bowel syndrome may be alleviated as well. Meditation is not a replacement for medical treatment, but it may prove a beneficial addition.

ASTHMA

Meditation can't cure asthma, but regular practice can alleviate symptoms and reduce their severity. Stress can trigger inflammation. Meditation lowers stress hormones and decreases activity in the body's sympathetic nervous system. Being more in control of these responses equates to better health. The deep breathing techniques used in meditation improve lung airflow.

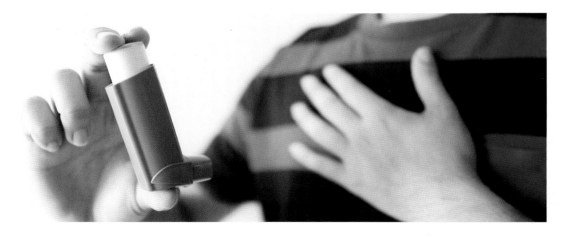

PAIN RELIEF

Some studies suggest that meditation activates parts of the brain in response to pain. One study noted that mindfulness meditation helped control pain without tapping the brain's own opiates. This conclusion suggests that it may be useful to combine meditation with pain medications to help manage a condition.

Another study focused on the use of mindfulness-based stress reduction training and cognitive-behavioral therapy to alleviate chronic lower back pain. Participants using these methods experienced greater improvement than those who received typical allopathic care.

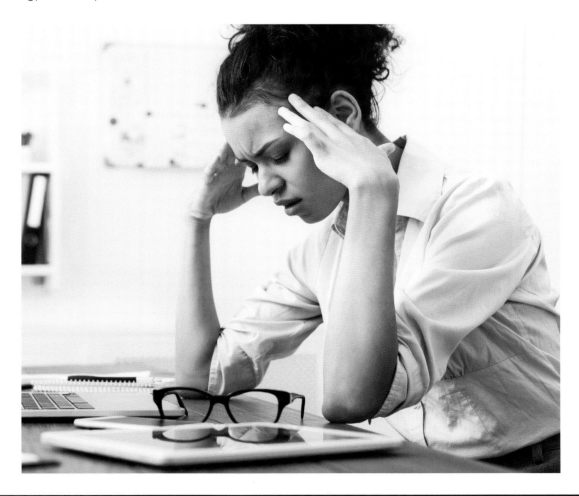

HIGH BLOOD PRESSURE

Studies suggest that practicing Transcendental Meditation may lower the risk of developing high blood pressure in those who have an increased risk of developing the condition. The American Heart Association has stated that evidence supports the use of this practice to lower blood pressure.

IRRITABLE BOWEL SYNDROME

There aren't a large number of studies to draw from, but at least one study found that meditation helped improve pain and quality of life in IBS sufferers. Another study noted that meditation muted the expression of genes related to inflammation and immune response, resulting in improved disease-related symptoms and anxiety. The key component of meditation that leads to these results seems to be the relaxation response.

The Relaxation Response

Simply put, this is the opposite of your body's fight-or-flight response. The term was coined by Dr. Herbert Benson, after observing the effects of meditation on the body. The response is typically defined as a person's ability to compel the body to relax—to release chemicals in the brain that bring about a physical state of deep rest.

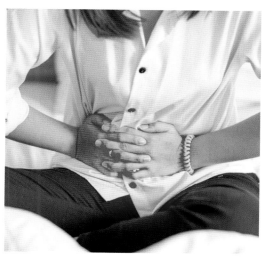

ANXIETY, DEPRESSION, AND INSOMNIA

Evidence suggests a link between mindfulness meditation and reduced anxiety and depression. One small study found a tangible link between the practice of mindfulness-based stress reduction and the reduction of insomnia severity in adults with chronic insomnia.

Beyond this though, an incredible amount of historical and anecdotal observation points to the fact that people who meditate regularly sleep better. It appears that regular meditation remolds or optimizes brain function in a way that allows for deeper, more restful sleep.

Depression affects about 20% of adults over 65. This condition can affect the body, leading to higher risks for heart disease and the severity of other illnesses. Incorporating meditation into daily life counteracts depression—it even changes brain regions linked to depression. So meditation is something like a rewiring process that fixes faulty circuits in the brain.

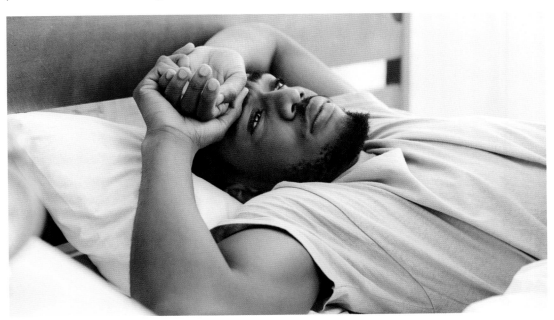

COGNITION

Meditation and mindfulness training may improve cognitive abilities. In addition to improved mood and emotional balance, meditation improves visuo-spatial processing, working memory, executive functioning, and increases attention span.

In one study, functional magnetic resonance imaging (fMRI) was used to scan brain activity in participants before and after they began regularly meditating. The scans revealed decreased activity in the amygdala when participants watched images with emotional content. The practice of meditation seemed to help them curb the involuntary emotional responses associated with this part of the brain.

Those who meditate regularly typically report an increased ability to perform tasks requiring focus. Even brief, 10-minute meditation sessions help the brain ward off distractions and concentrate on the task at hand.

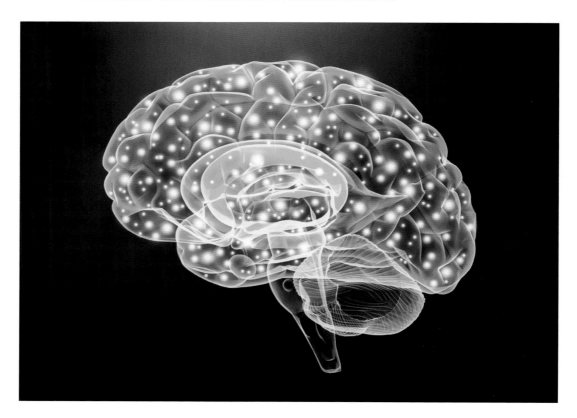

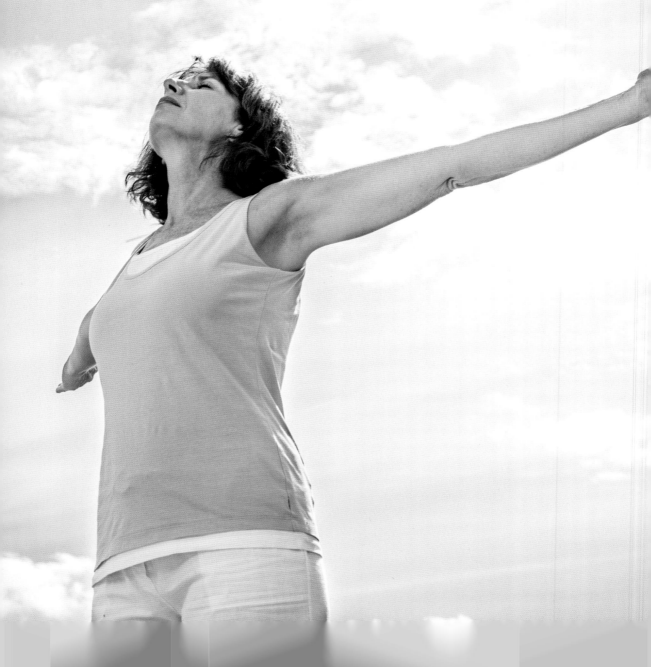

JUST BREATHE

ANAPANASATI

The word *Anapanasati* translates to "mindfulness of breathing." This form of meditation was taught by the founder of Buddhism, Gautama Buddha. His teachings about mindfulness in relation to inhalation and exhalation are found in the Anapanasati Sutta. According to these teachings, the practice reveals the link between body and mind. It is also considered a foundation or gateway to subsequent meditation practices, and it was the first subject of meditation the Buddha addressed.

Regardless of where your meditation practice takes you, you will always return to breathing and mindfulness of the act of breathing. Total concentration on inhalation and exhalation will lead you squarely into the present moment. Breathe!

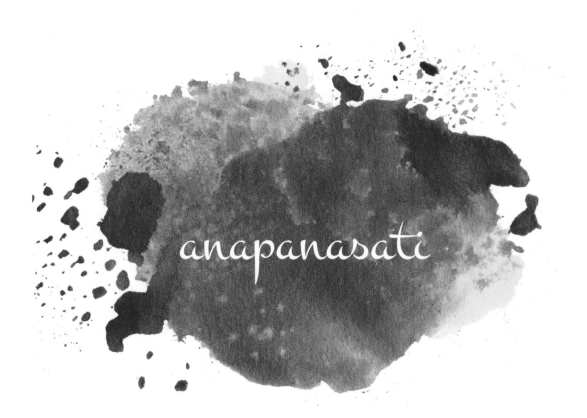

anapanasati

There is one way of breathing that is shameful and constricted. Then, there's another way: a breath of love that takes you all the way to infinity.

—Rumi

Meditative breathing is a great entry point for a meditation beginner. It's a challenge to practice, but it's simple to learn. Breath exercises can be just part of a larger practice, such as Vipassana or Zazen. They can also be the whole heart and soul of a practice.

Time
The length of your breathing practice depends on the method you use and what you're using it for.

Posture
You can sit or stand in a comfortable position, or hold another pose when doing a movement meditation.

Remember
Your mind will wander, and that's ok. That's part of what you're working on with this type of meditation. When your mind wanders or becomes fixed on a topic, acknowledge that it has. Then gently bring your attention back to your breath.

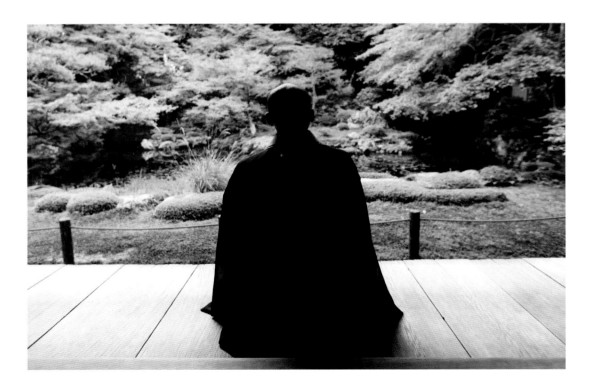

BREATH AWARENESS

Spend a few minutes with simple breath awareness to ground yourself before beginning another meditation practice, or spend a longer time with it as a mindfulness exercise.

All you have to do is bring your attention to your breath. Breathe naturally; there's no need to lengthen or shorten your inhales or exhales.

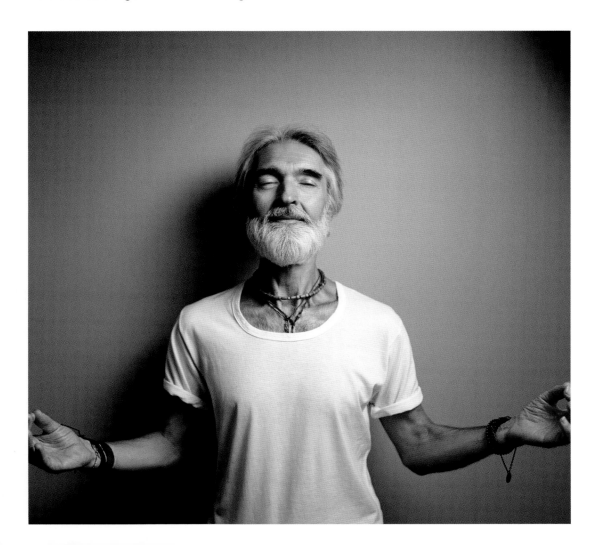

BELLY BREATHING

This is a good technique to use throughout your practice. It involves deliberate control of your diaphragm, the muscle located just below the lungs. Contracting the diaphragm makes space for the lungs to expand and take in air. The diaphragm relaxes as you exhale.

To prepare, place one palm flat against your chest. Place the other palm just below your ribs, the location of your diaphragm. Inhale slowly, letting your belly expand out as the diaphragm contracts. Your chest should remain more or less unchanged. Then exhale slowly. Let your belly come back down as the diaphragm relaxes. Again, your chest should remain more or less unchanged.

BREATH COUNTING

Use this to help ground yourself if your mind has been wandering uncontrollably during a meditation session, or if you just need a moment of focus and clarity during the day.

Count each inhale and exhale (inhale 1, exhale 2, inhale 3, exhale 4, and so on) until you reach 6. Then start again from 1.

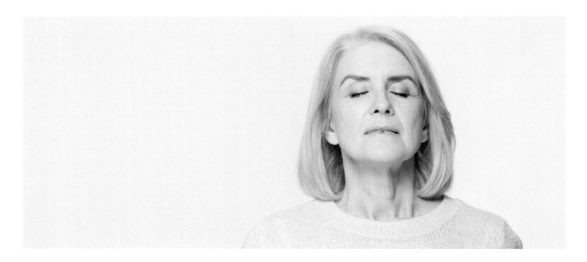

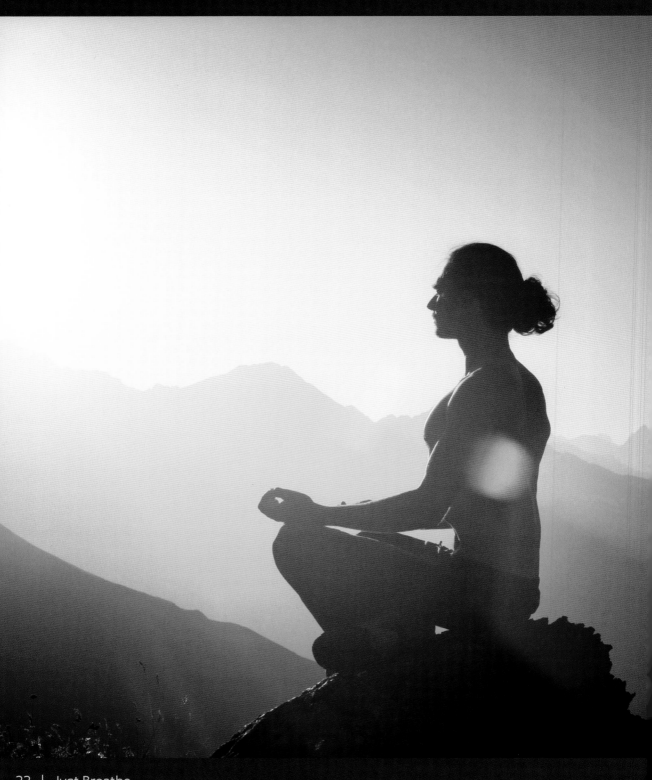

4-7-8 BREATHING

A few cycles of this exercise can help calm your nerves. Some insomniacs also find it helps them fall asleep.

Inhale through your nose for a count of 4, filling your lungs. Pause for a count of 7. Exhale through your mouth for a count of 8, emptying your lungs. Then repeat the cycle.

4-COUNT BREATHING

Use this exercise as a stand-alone meditation or as part of a larger practice.

Inhale for a count of 4. Pause for a count of 4. Exhale for a count of 4. Pause for a count of 4. Then repeat the cycle.

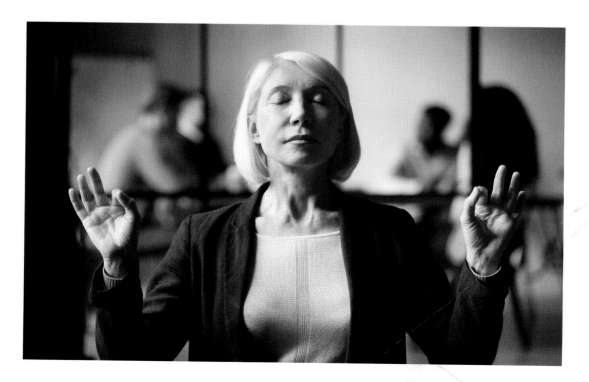

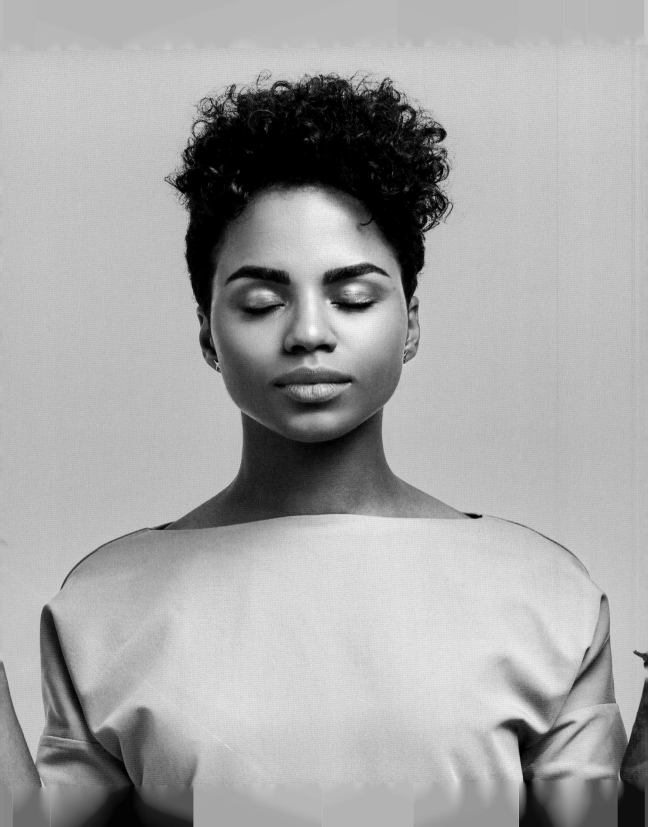

BELLOWS BREATH

Bring energy to your body and alertness to your mind with this stimulating technique. Start small with this exercise, with each inhale/exhale cycle lasting a full second. Increase the speed of the cycles gradually, as your comfort allows.

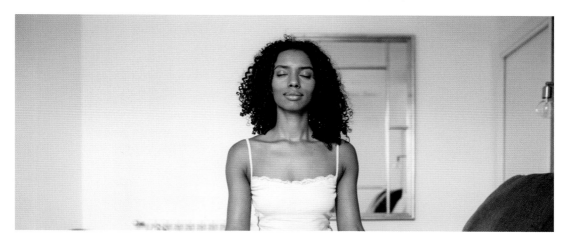

HOW TO DO IT

Step 1
Inhale and exhale sharply through the nose in quick succession for 10 seconds. Breathe from the diaphragm, as in belly breathing.

Step 2
Rest for 30 seconds, breathing naturally.

Step 3
Return to your quick bellows breath for 20 seconds. Then rest for another 30 seconds.

Step 4
Return to bellows breath for 30 seconds. Then breathe naturally.

TECHNIQUES TO RELIEVE STRESS

Breathing exercises can bring down stress levels without requiring large investments of time. You can begin with five minutes a day and increase the duration as time permits.

Alternate nostril breathing lowers the heart rate and relaxes the body. You should be comfortably seated when practicing this technique.
- Press your right nostril closed and inhale through your left nostril.
- Press your left nostril closed and exhale through your right nostril.
- Inhale through your right nostril and then close this nostril.
- Exhale through your left nostril.

Repeat this cycle for about five minutes.

Equal breathing focuses on creating a balance between inhaling and exhaling. This balancing technique enhances mental balance. Breathe in and out through your nose. Count during each inhale and exhale, giving each one equal time. You can incorporate a slight pause after each inhale and exhale if this feels comfortable. Repeat this cycle for about five minutes.

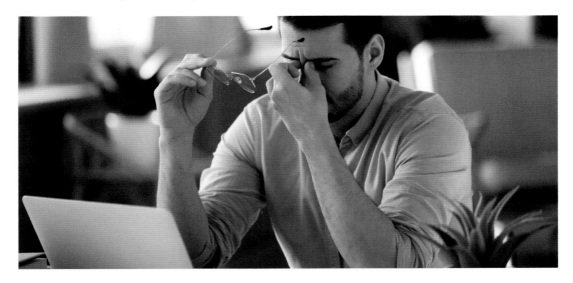

Resonant breathing (also known as coherent breathing) reduces stress and maximizes your heart rate variability. This technique imposes a rate of five full breaths (both inhales and exhales) per minute. To do this, simply count to five as you inhale and count to five as you exhale. Do this for several minutes.

Breath focus uses words to assist relaxation. Choose a word or phrase that has positive or neutral connotations for you. Sit comfortably and try the following for ten minutes:

- Focus on your natural breathing without changing it.
- While continuing to focus on your breath, bring up the word or phrase and begin repeating it silently.
- Imagine that the air you breathe in is full of peace and calm.
- Imagine that the air you exhale is carrying away the stress, like a wave going out to sea.

Pursed lip breathing makes you slow down the pace of your breathing. Relax your neck and shoulders as much as possible. Inhale slowly through your nose for two counts. Purse your lips as if you were going to whistle and exhale through them for four counts.

Deep breathing is particularly effective for shortness of breath. It moves more fresh air into your lungs while helping you to relax and feel more balanced. You may stand or sit for this technique

- Pull your elbows back slightly.
- Inhale deeply through your nose.
- Hold your breath for five counts.
- Slowly exhale through your nose.

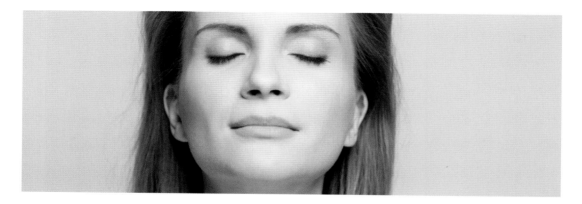

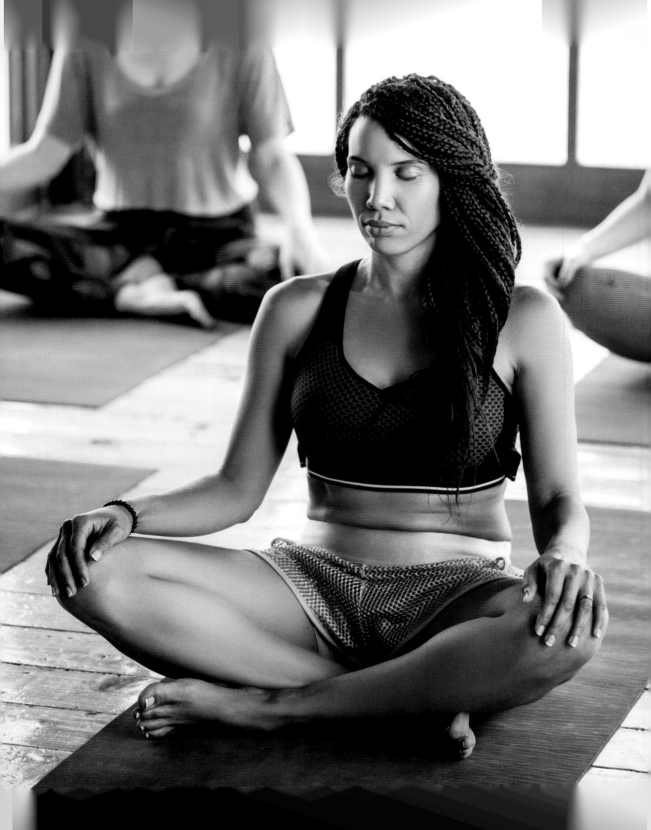

By all means use sometimes to be alone.

Salute thyself: see what thy soul doth wear.

Dare to look in thy chest; for 't is thine own;

And tumble up and down what thou find'st there.

Who cannot rest till he good fellows finde,

He breaks up house, turns out of doores his minde.

—George Herbert

THE STRESS RESPONSE

Traffic congestion, arguments, public speaking, financial worries, deadlines—everyone has triggers that lead to stress responses. The body's stress response is natural and hardwired into us. It is not a fault or a defect. It involves an accelerated heart rate and the diversion of blood away from the gut and into the muscles. It constricts our pupils. It alters our breathing. This is the body preparing itself for running away or engaging in conflict—fight or flight.

The hypothalamus is tied to the stress response. It is connected to the body through the autonomic nervous system. It releases hormones into the body which, if present for too long, result in the adrenal glands releasing cortisol. This hormone can negatively affect the immune system's ability to do its job. Chronic stress is associated with abnormalities in stress hormones and inflammatory markers. It increases blood pressure and raises the risk of heart attacks and strokes. Increased levels of cortisol are linked to weight gain as well.

The stress response can be countered. Meditation and breathing techniques offer a way to *retrain* the body's response to stressful situations. Whereas rapid breathing is controlled by the sympathetic nervous system, deliberately slow and deep breathing stimulates an opposing parasympathetic reaction of "rest and digest."

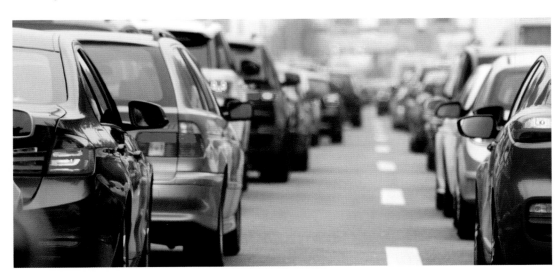

BRAIN AND BODY

The fact that we can retrain our bodies to respond to stress in a less negative way is truly remarkable. Research has demonstrated that breathing techniques can change gene expression. In other words, we have the power to alter the basic activity of our cells with our minds. And long-term meditation seems to increase the amount of the brain's gray matter in the auditory and sensory cortex. In other words, your senses become enhanced. Gray matter also increases in the frontal cortex, a region associated with memory and executive decision making.

In one study, researchers found that people who meditated for only eight weeks had modified their brains in several areas. While the amygdala had shrunk, other regions thickened. These included the posterior cingulate, the left hippocampus, the temporal parietal junction, and the Pons. So while meditation is changing the brain, the brain is also changing the body. With such a powerful and free tool at our disposal, why wouldn't we meditate?

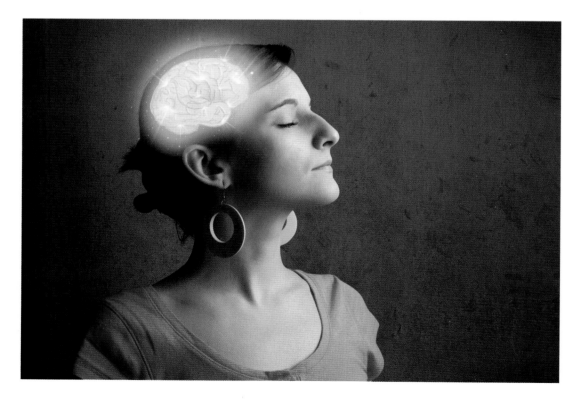

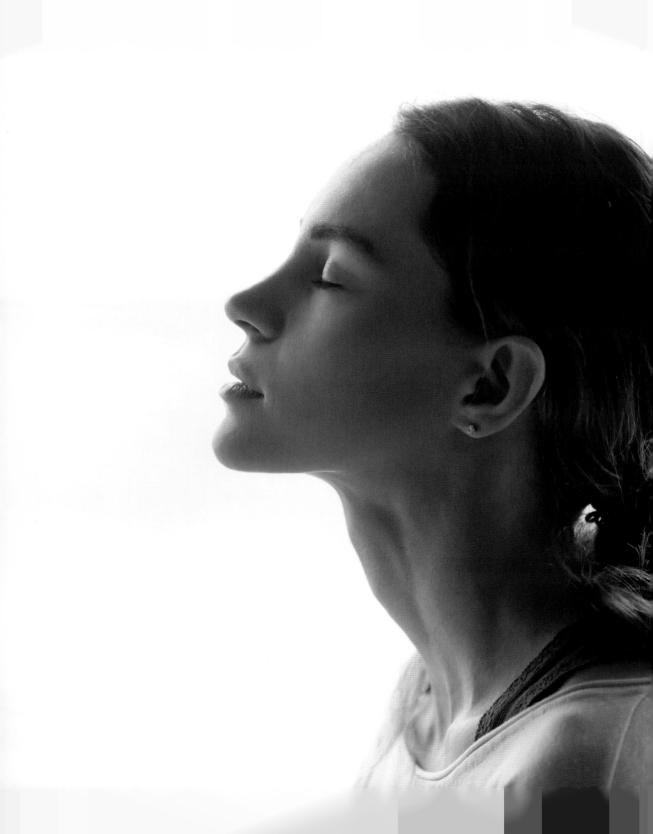

When the breath wanders, the mind also is unsteady. But when the breath is calmed the mind too will be still, and the yogi achieves long life. Therefore, one should learn to control the breath.

—Hatha Yoga Pradipika

As long as there is breath in the body, there is life. When breath departs, so too does life. Therefore, regulate the breath.

—Hatha Yoga Pradipika

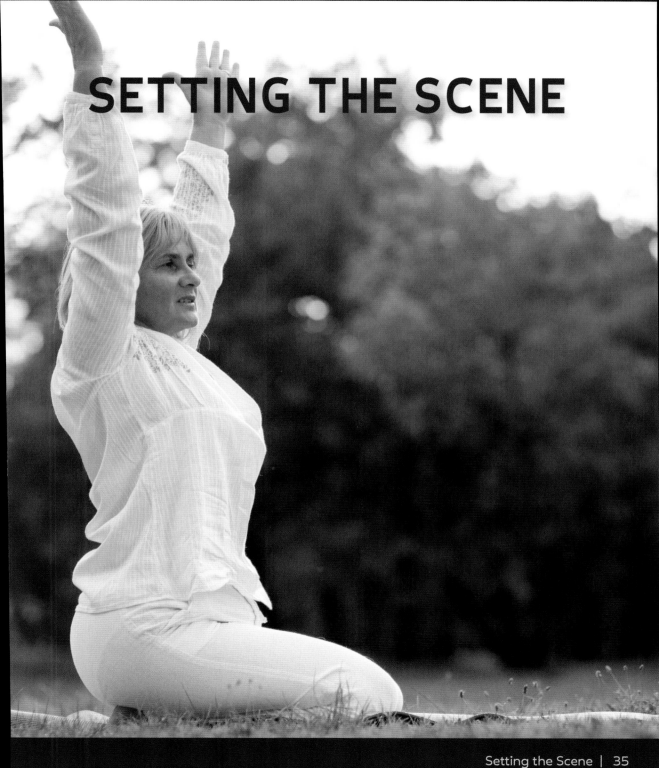

SETTING THE SCENE

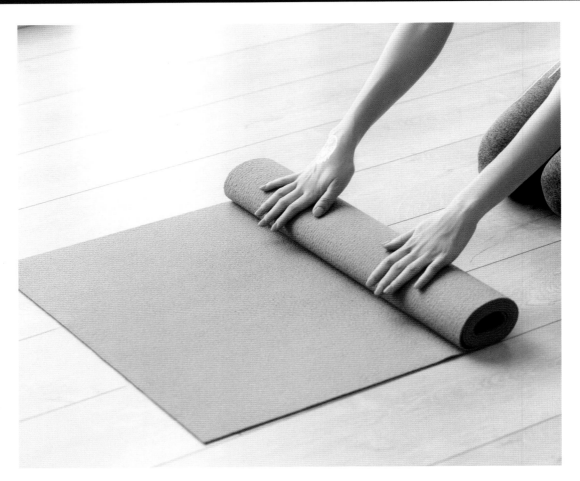

THE RIGHT SETTING

Creating the right setting can help set the right tone for your meditation practice. Keep in mind what the demands of your chosen meditation technique are. Will you be sitting for a long time? Is movement or balance involved? How much space will you need? How much time?

Getting everything right can take some experimentation. As you try one setup or another out, you might be surprised at what ends up working or not working. Plus, sometimes elements you thought you needed can prove to be unnecessary, or vice versa.

TIME AND PLACE

Choosing a Time

When do you want to meditate? Find a time that could ideally work for you in the long term. Some people swear by morning meditation so they can start the day with clarity and awareness. Others have an easier time meditating later in the day, as they unwind and reflect on the day's events. Whenever you practice, set aside a specific block of time before you begin, whether it's five minutes or two hours.

Try this:

In the morning

- First thing, shortly after waking
- Around a simple morning routine such as making coffee or brushing your teeth, meditating during the activity
- During the commute to school or work

In the afternoon

- During your lunch break
- As you run errands

In the evening

- Right after returning home from school or work
- Shortly before bed

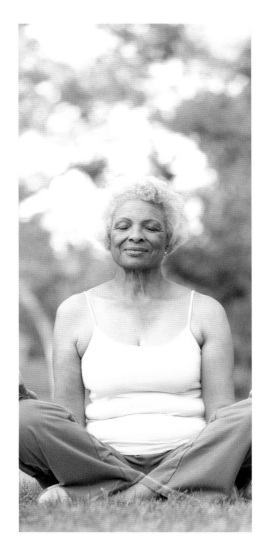

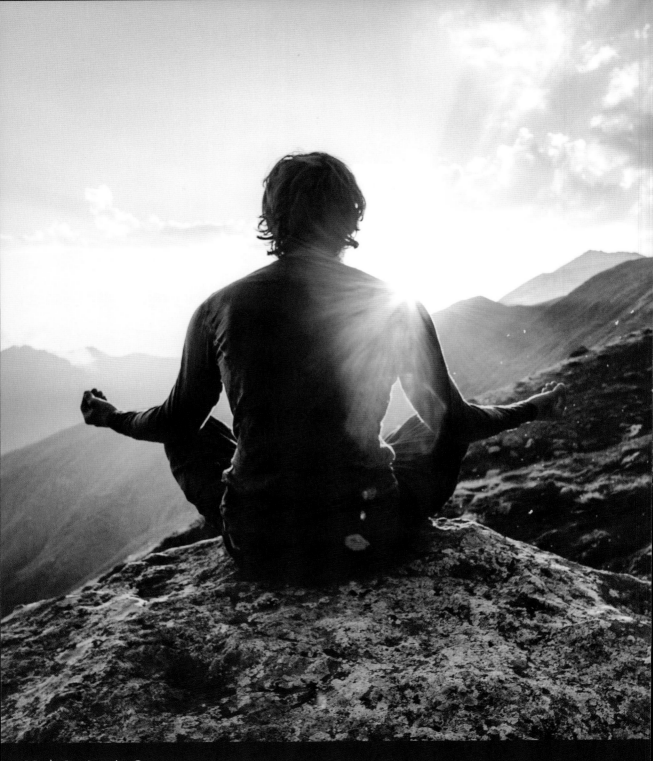

CHOOSING A PLACE

You could do most types of meditation just about anywhere. If you're able to, however, look for a place you can visit regularly, where there are few distractions, and where you feel safe and comfortable.

You can also set aside a location solely for meditation, whose appearance, smell, and feel you'll come to associate with meditation. This can improve your practice and help you turn it into a regular habit.

A few places to try:

At home

- A corner or small area with enough space to meditate
- Backyard
- Separate room

In Public

- Park
- Library
- Place of worship

With a community

- Classes in meditation
- Regular meetings with friends or colleagues

Extra Practice

Sometimes you need a mental tune-up in addition to your regular practice. A brief meditation can help you bring calm awareness to any number of situations, from daily annoyances to nerve-wracking moments. To name just a few:

- While waiting in line
- While stuck in traffic
- When a stressful deadline is closing in
- Before giving a speech or presentation
- Before a game or competition
- Before a difficult conversation

PROPS

Props help you maintain comfort and ease in your body, particularly when you're in a seated position or a yoga pose. When meditating, you often remain in the same position for an extended period of time, and you should be able to remain (more or less) focused inward with as few bodily distractions as possible. Therefore, comfort is paramount.

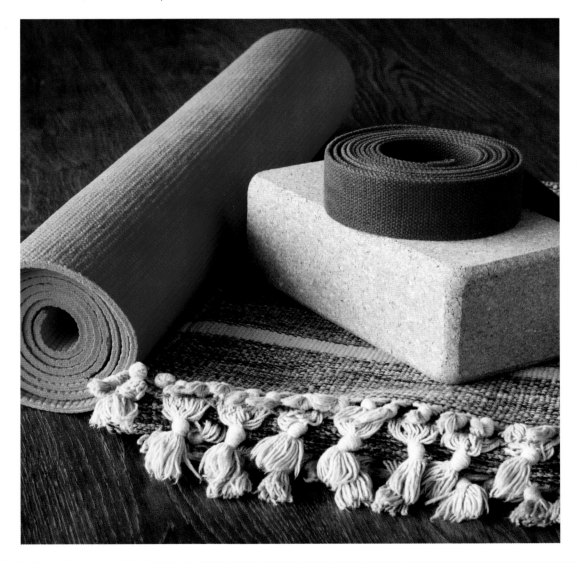

Support

Many of us struggle with staying comfortable in an erect seated position, with our backs straight and necks long. Sometimes the issue is flexibility around the hips, lower back, or knees; sometimes it's strength; and sometimes it's another issue entirely. Whatever the cause, sitting—especially low to the floor—can be a challenge. One way to solve this is to sit on something to raise our hips a little higher. This makes it easier for you to sit up straight.

Meditation Cushions

Firm, round meditation cushions are called zafus or putuans. They're most often used in seated meditations. People generally use these cushions when sitting cross-legged on the floor.

Zabutons are square cushions that are usually thinner and softer than zafus or bolsters. They're often used as extra cushioning underneath zafus or when kneeling.

There are also heart- and crescent-shaped cushions. You can find cushions in a range of heights. As a general rule, the less flexible your hips, lower back, or knees are, the higher your cushion should be.

Bolsters

Bolsters tend to be longer than meditation cushions, and may be either rectangular or cylindrical. They are great when you need some extra support under your hips, knees, or other body part when sitting or lying down.

Lumbar Support

If you're sitting with your back against the wall or the back of a chair, extra support at the small of your back can help you comfortably maintain good posture. Small lumbar pillows are designed precisely for this.

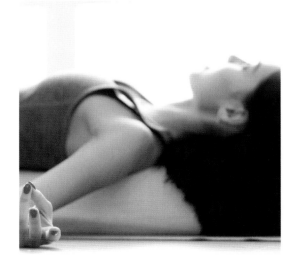

Blocks

If you're kneeling, you can place a block under your hip bones, between your knees. This provides a little extra height to reduce the stress on your knees.

Blocks are also handy when you want to enter a yoga pose but need support under your hands, knees, or another part of your body in order to make the position accessible.

Find a kind of block whose firmness suits your needs. Foam blocks are generally the softest. Cork blocks are harder, and wood blocks even harder.

Benches and Chairs

Meditation benches can make kneeling more comfortable. The seats are tilted forward. This puts your hips in the right position to support good posture. The benches are just tall and wide enough to fit your feet and ankles underneath when you kneel. There are also specialty meditation chairs. These keep you low to the ground but also support your back.

Meditation Mat

The ground can be hard and slippery. In these situations, adding an extra layer between you and the ground can be a good idea.

Yoga Mat

Yoga mats can be used as cushioning, but they might be better at providing a grippy surface. This is particularly important when you're attempting poses that require secure foot or hand placement.

Easy Alternatives

You don't have to buy special equipment if you need some extra support for your meditation. You can always use items around the house instead, such as:

- Books
- Pillows
- Blankets
- Chairs
- Chair cushions

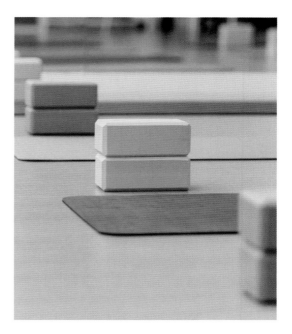

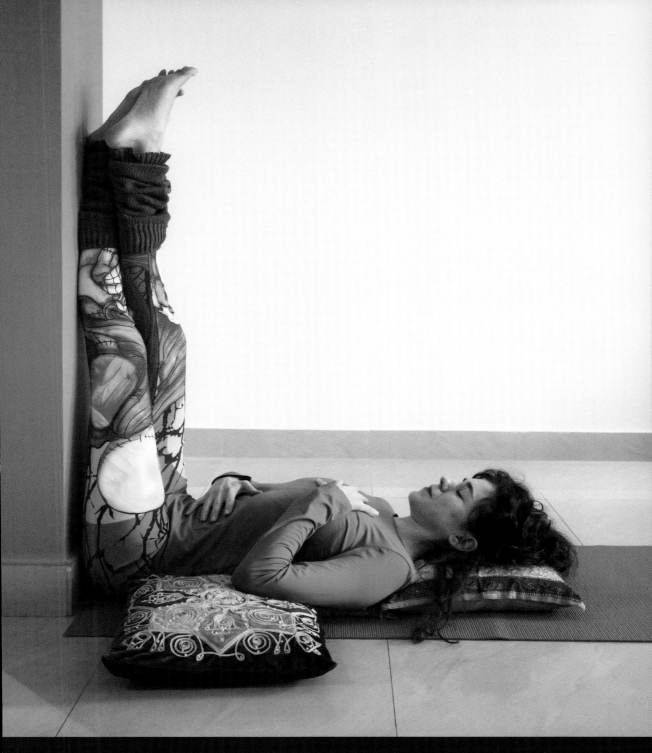

SCENTS AND SOUNDS

Scents

A scent can affect your mood, even when you're not consciously paying attention to it. With this in mind, you can change the atmosphere of your meditation space dramatically by adding certain scents. Incense, essential oils, candles, and a variety of other sources are just a few examples of how to accomplisth this.

Neroli

A product of bitter orange blossoms, neroli oil is used to inspire cheerfulness, enthusiasm, mental clarity, and creativity.

Benzoin

The scent, produced by benzoin resin, can produce a feeling of stability, comfort, and groundedness.

Cardamom

Cardamom's spicy smell is known to increase blood flow to the brain. It can also bring greater alertness, clarity, self-worth, and inspiration.

Cedarwood

This scent actually comes from a juniper tree, not cedar. Its scent can help a person access inner strength and self-reliance, as well as better judgement skills.

Bitter Orange

While bitter orange flowers produce neroli, the fruit's rind produces bitter orange oil. This and other citrus scents are uplifting, and they can bring relaxation and patience.

Vetiver

This comes from vetiver grass. Its scent combats mental fatigue and anxiety. It can also improve a person's breathing during sleep.

Lavender

The flowers of the lavender plant are as pleasing to the eye as they are to the nose. Lavender is well-known for its relaxing smell.

Sandalwood

The sandalwood tree produces a heady-scented wood. The smell can reduce anxiety even as it increases alertness.

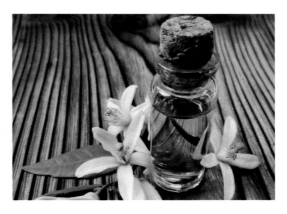

DIFFUSION

Diffusers are small electrical units that release a mist of essential oil vapor into a room. Nebulizers also pump essential oil vapor into the air, but do it without water. Generally, you place a few drops of essential oil in a glass container and turn on a small compressor that's connected with a piece of tubing. The unit disperses a fine mist of micro-particles mixed with the stream of air produced by the pump. This method increases the surface area of the molecules. Clay and terra cotta discs and holders are simple and cheap. Add a few drops of oil to the disc surface and allow natural sunlight to heat up the surface and disperse the scent.

Blends

You can customize oil blends for your own meditation needs. Simply combine the oils with water in a diffuser. Here are a few ideas.

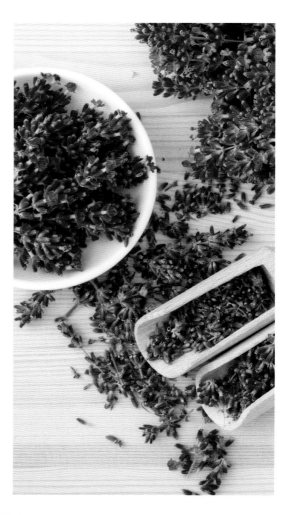

Relaxation blend:
- 4 drops lavender oil
- 3 drops clary sage oil
- 2 drops ylang ylang oil
- 1 drop marjoram oil

Tranquil evening blend:
- 3 drops lavender oil
- 3 drops vetiver oil
- 3 drops frankincense oil

Attention and focus blend:
- 2 drops grapefruit oil
- 2 drops lavender oil
- 2 drops lemon oil
- 2 drops peppermint oil
- 1 drop basil oil
- 1 drop rosemary oil

Sound

Another way to personalize your meditation space is with sound. Experiment to find what best suits your practice; some sounds might be calming or entrancing, while others are just distracting.

Ambient Music

This music is designed to be in the background. You might associate this kind of instrumental music with elevators, but it can also be useful in meditation. It can affect the way you feel without making many demands on your attention.

Chants

Chants are a feature in many religions around the world. Listening to them can help quieten your mind and help you focus.

Instrumental Tones

Gongs, bells, chimes, and digeridoo sounds can calm your mind, or give you something to focus on.

Singing Bowls

A singing bowl is a type of bell that has long been used in Buddhist meditation. You play it by rubbing a mallet around the bowl's outside rim. This produces a clear, constant tone. You can either listen to recordings of singing bowls or play one yourself.

Nature Sounds

There are countless types of nature sounds that can fill your space. Recordings of rain, thunder, or beach waves can be easy to find. There are also a range of animal sounds, from birdsong, to whale song, and various things in between.

Binaural Beats

These are tones, sometimes accompanied by music, that you listen to through headphones. One ear hears one tone, and the other ear hears a tone at a slightly different frequency. As a result of the difference in frequency, you hear a completely new, pulsing tone.

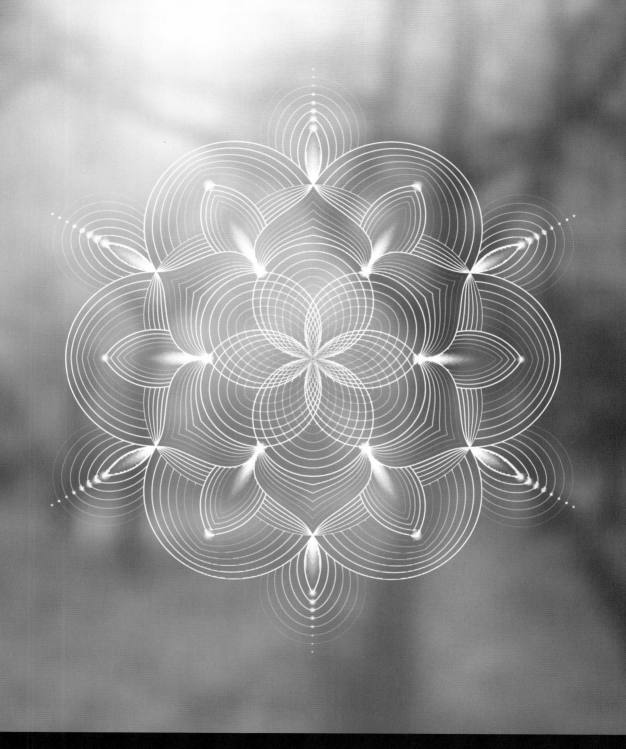

OTHER CONSIDERATIONS

As simple as meditation sometimes seems, putting it into practice can be a challenge. Keep the ideas below in mind as you begin your practice. They can help make the start a little easier.

The goal of meditation is simple and singular: to meditate. That's it. There is no need to worry about anything else as you practice.

Meditation does not need to be perfect. It is continual practice. Everyone has easier days and more difficult days. Be kind to yourself—to try is really to succeed.

Your mind will wander. When it does, take a moment to notice what it is that has distracted you. Then gently bring your attention back to the focus of your meditation.

Let thoughts and emotions come and go. Don't try to suppress or remove them. Acknowledge them when they appear, and then let them go.

Wear comfortable clothing. Yoga leggings or loose pants, fitted tank or oversized sweater—whatever keeps you comfortable, wear that. Soft fabrics are a good idea, as are outfits that allow freedom of movement.

No method works for everyone. Each of us has a unique brain and body. Find what works for your brain and body. Experiment and explore.

Decide how long you want to meditate before you begin. Start small, perhaps with a 3- to 4-minute meditation. As you become more comfortable with the practice, you can increase the time.

A timer can make a huge difference. You don't want to keep breaking your concentration to look at your watch. Set an alarm on your phone or even use an egg timer.

Make meditation a routine. As much as possible, meditate at the same time and in the same place each time you practice. This makes it easier to keep the practice up over time.

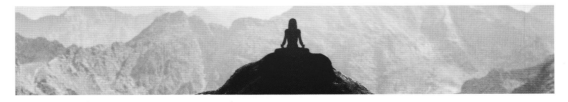

How often you meditate matters more than how long you meditate. Set aside time to practice at least a couple of days a week. Work toward practicing every day if you can, even if it's only for a few minutes at a time.

Meditation involves your entire self, positive and negative. Difficult emotions surface as easily as positive ones. If you have trouble with negative thoughts as you meditate, perhaps try talking with a professional who is either a counselor or an expert in that form of meditation.

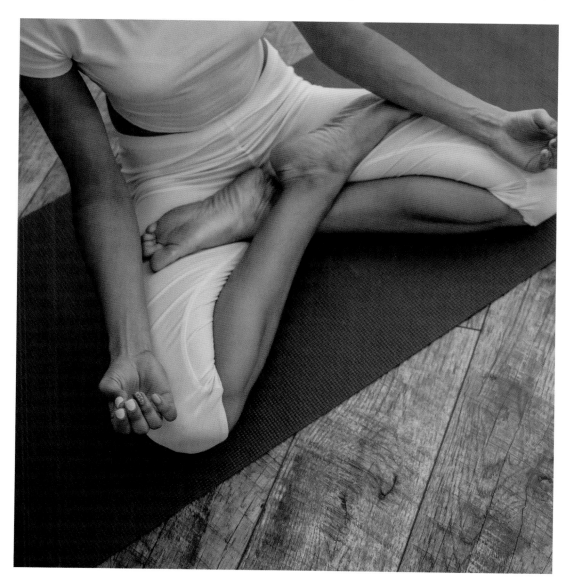

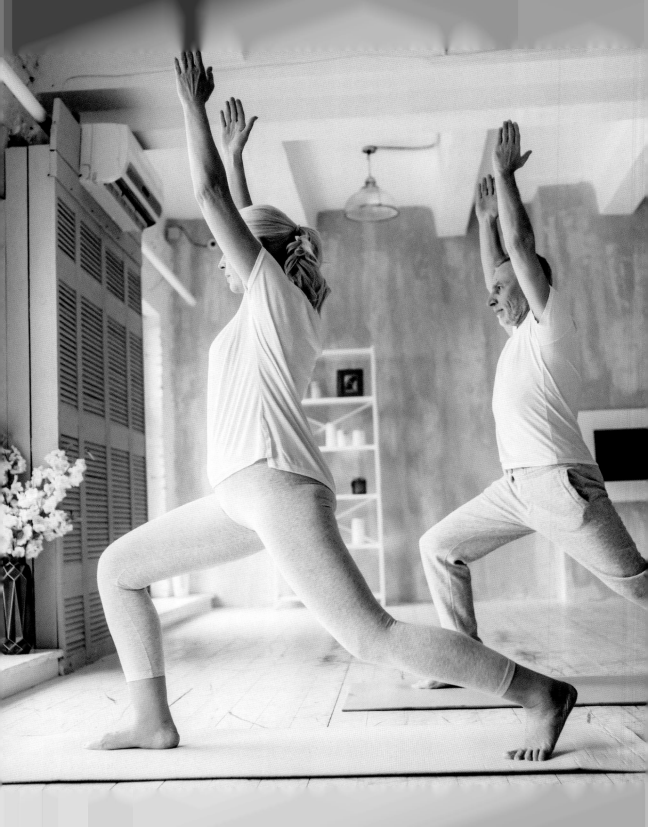

Concentration helps us to withdraw our scattered minds from different directions. The mind has been scattered. It wanders among various objects, which are impressions in our minds. The mind has been divided, and thus mental energy is dissipated. Very little energy is left for the accomplishment of the real ideals in life. But gradually we learn by concentration how to withdraw the scattered forces of the mind and how to focus them.

—Swami Vivekananda

The mind is subject to moods, as the shadows of clouds pass over the earth. Pay not too much heed to them. Let not the traveler stop for them.

—Henry David Thoreau

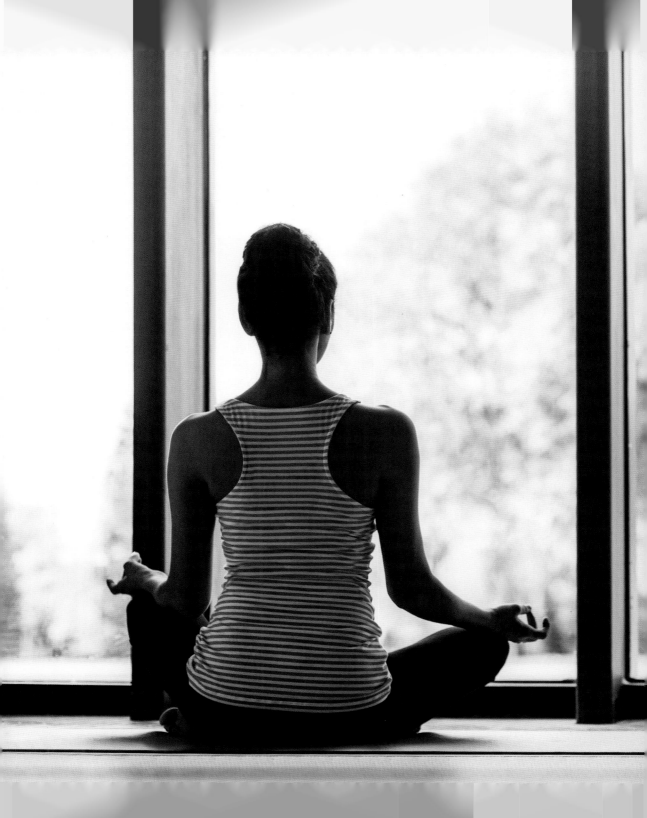

MEDITATIONS

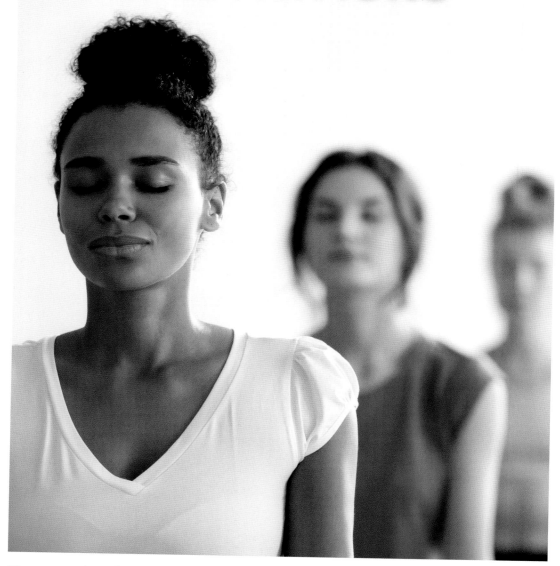

There are a lot of meditation techniques out there, with a variety of focuses and intentions. The methods described in this book are some of the most common or well-known. If you don't know where to start, turn the page and take a look at the cheat sheet for some ideas.

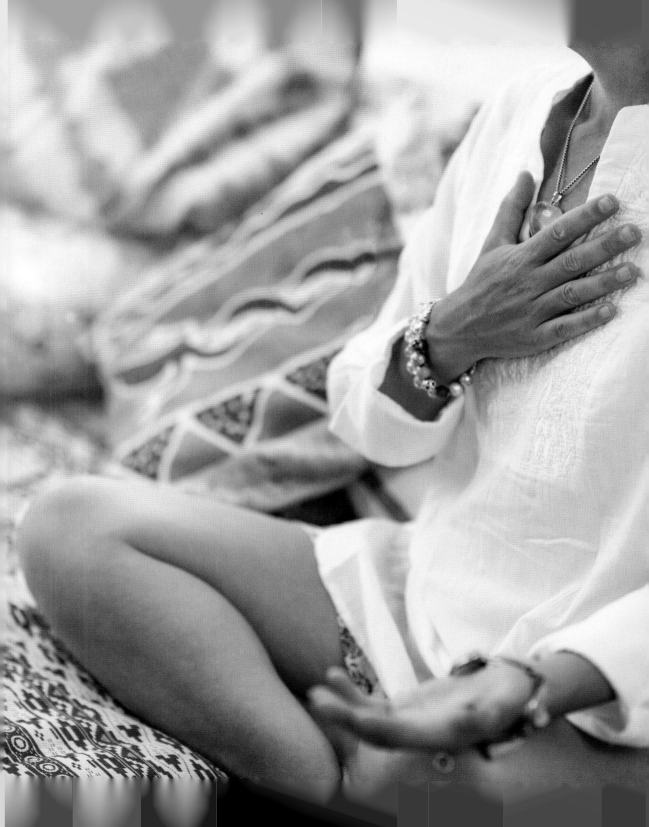

CHEAT SHEET

Not sure where to start with meditation? These categories might help.

Internal Focus

- Chakra
- Metta
- Mindfulness
- Noting
- Self-reflection
- Meditation
- Third Eye
- Vipassana
- Zazen

External Focus

- Gazing
- Mantras
- Sound

Body-focused

- Body Scan
- Breathing Meditation
- Heartbeat Meditation
- Progressive Muscle Relaxation
- Walking Meditation

Movement

- Dancing Meditation
- Qigong
- Walking Meditation
- Whirling
- Yoga

Creative

- Art Meditation
- Dancing Meditation

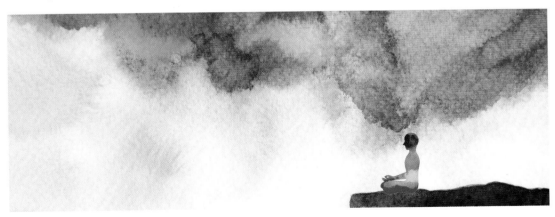

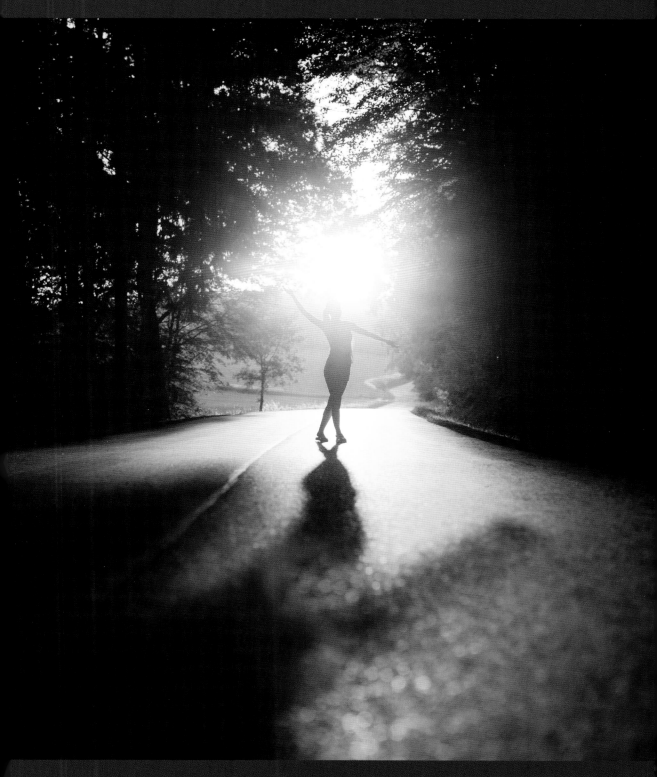

Watch your thoughts; they become words. Watch your words; they become actions. Watch your actions; they become habits. Watch your habits; they become character. Watch your character; for it becomes your destiny.

—the Upanishads

It is good to tame the mind, which is difficult to hold in and flighty, rushing wherever it listeth; a tamed mind brings happiness.

—the Dhammapada

ART MEDITATION

Art can help a busy mind become calm. Mandalas are a great example. Sand mandalas made in some schools of Buddhism are intricately-patterned, circular creations of dyed sands. Completing one is a days-long endeavor that creators use as a method of disciplined meditation. Once complete, the mandala is destroyed as a representation of the impermanence of all things. Some Buddhists make or use painted, drawn, or other permanent mandalas. With these, a person uses their experience of the art as meditation, focusing on the structure, pattern, and symbolism the images contain.

Meditative art is not limited to mandalas. If you're creating something, it can look like anything, and be made with whatever art supplies you like. If you choose to observe art, the art can be anything that draws you in.

Either way, your focus is on what is before you. Give all your attention to what you are doing, seeing, feeling, smelling, or (depending on the art) tasting. This pointed concentration can lead to greater calmness, clarity, and relaxation.

Time
If you're just starting out, try meditating for 5 to 10 minutes. You can increase the length of time as you become more comfortable.

Remember
Your mind will wander, and that's ok. When it wanders, acknowledge that it has. Then gently bring your attention back to the art.

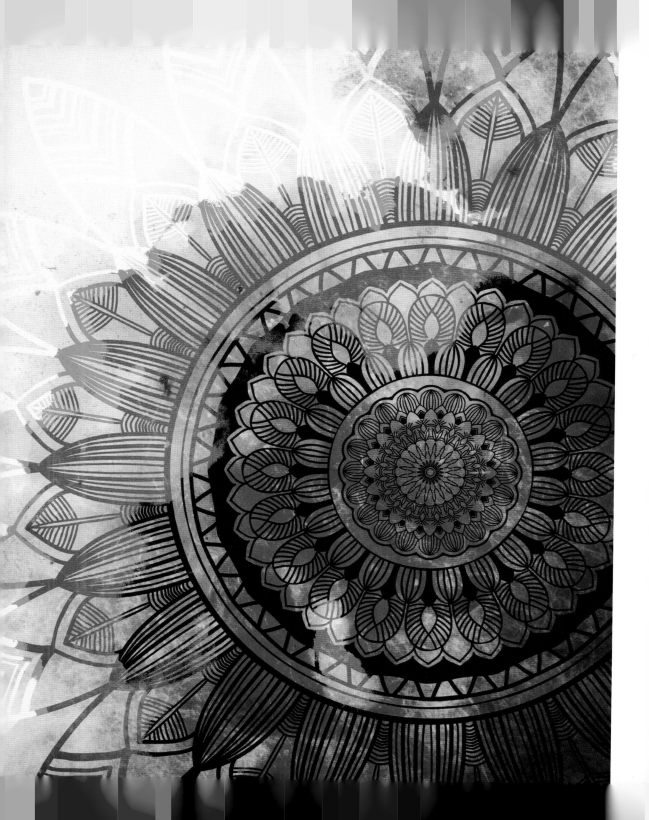

CREATING ART

Creating art as part of your meditation is not an exercise in making "good" art. Try to avoid passing judgement on your work. Focus on the process, rather than the product.

You can have a freeform sort of meditation by creating art purely by "feel." Start by taking a moment to simply focus on your breath. When you're ready, begin your creation. Move slowly if that suits you, move faster if that feels right. Focus on what you are doing—choosing a color, drawing a shape—in the moment. What you'll do next doesn't matter yet, and what you did before doesn't matter anymore. As thoughts appear, acknowledge them and let them fade.

If following a structure helps, try your hand at a mandala. You don't have to use sand; all you need is a piece of paper and something to draw with.

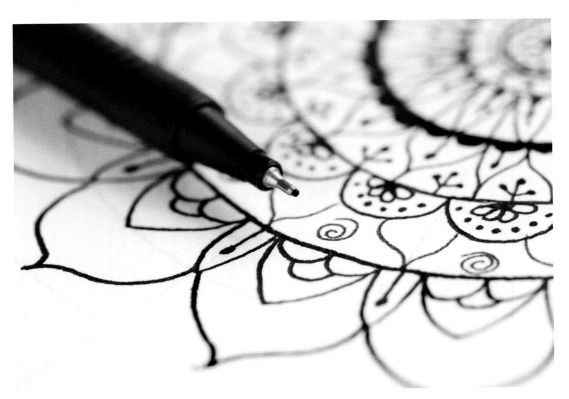

HOW TO DO IT

Step 1
Take a few deep breaths to ground yourself. Then return to natural breathing.

Step 2
Draw a small circle, perhaps a centimeter wide, in the center of the paper. This can be freehand or with a compass.

Step 3
Draw a repeating, symmetrical pattern in a ring around the circle. It could be a series of leaves that "grow" from the circle, a ring of dots that encircle it, or anything else. Take your time as you do it, noting the feeling of your hand as it draws, and seeing the shapes you create.

Step 4
Draw a different pattern in a ring around what you have so far. This, too, should be symmetrical, and completely encircle what you have so far.

Step 5
Continue adding rings, changing patterns, until you run out of space on the page.

Step 6 (optional)
You can color in your mandala after you finish drawing.

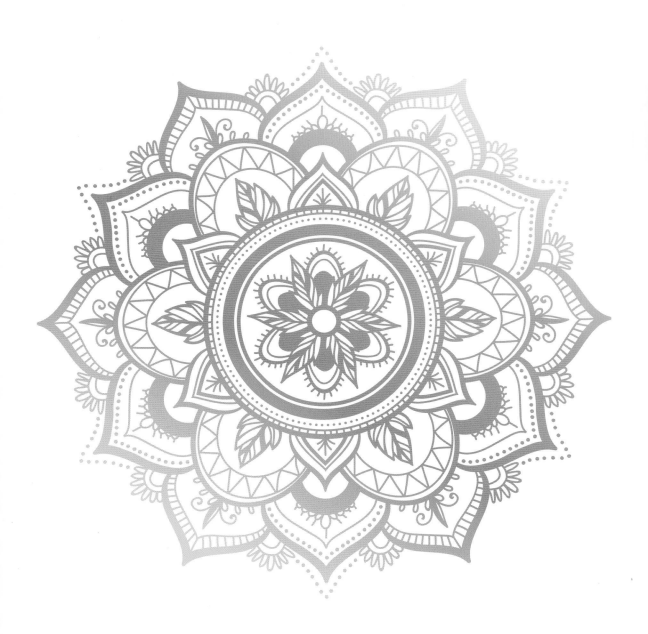

EXPERIENCING ART

Painting, sculpture, photograph, or clay pot, you can incorporate existing art into meditation. In this type of practice, your focus is on the sensations that come as you study the artwork.

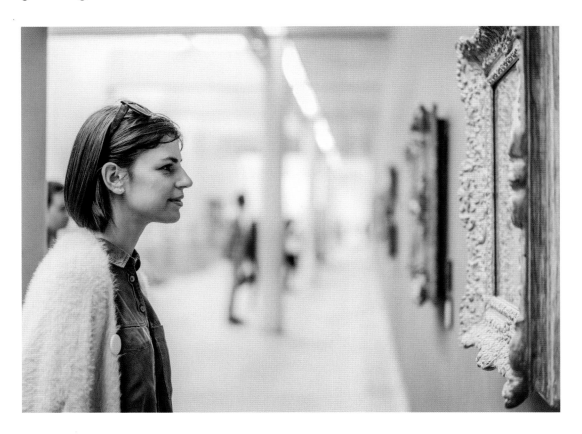

HOW TO DO IT

Step 1
Close your eyes and take a few deep breaths. Then return to normal breathing.

Step 2
Open your eyes and look at the image as a whole. Note any initial reactions you have to it, any emotions, thoughts, or memories it conjures.

Step 3
Consider the details of the image. What colors do you see? What shapes? What textures? How do objects or elements in the piece of art interact with one another?

Step 4
Imagine yourself becoming part of what you see in the artwork. You're in the setting of the the image. Go through your senses. What do you smell, hear, feel, taste? This can work even if the art is abstract; what sensations come to you when you imagine being inside or surrounded by the colors and shapes?

Step 5
When you're ready to end the meditation, close your eyes again and take a few deep breaths.

WABI-SABI

The artwork you consider during meditation doesn't have to be beautiful or perfect. You might find that contemplating an old, chipped coffee cup serves your purpose just as well. The Buddhist focus on the impermanence of life finds resonance in the Japanese concept of wabi-sabi. Life—and art—is fleeting and imperfect. Wabi-sabi finds beauty in this imperfection. It is the beauty of modest and humble things. Nothing lasts. Nothing is perfect. Accepting this opens the door to the perception of a deeper beauty. It's an aesthetic that opens the eyes to the growing, decaying, dying profundity of nature. Above all, it reveres authenticity.

Wabi-sabi parallels some of the ideas that naturally arise in the practice of meditation, like accepting the transience of things. One accepts that objects will wear and change as they are used. Suffering is linked to the damage and wear of life itself. Our use of a thing can define the thing itself for a moment.

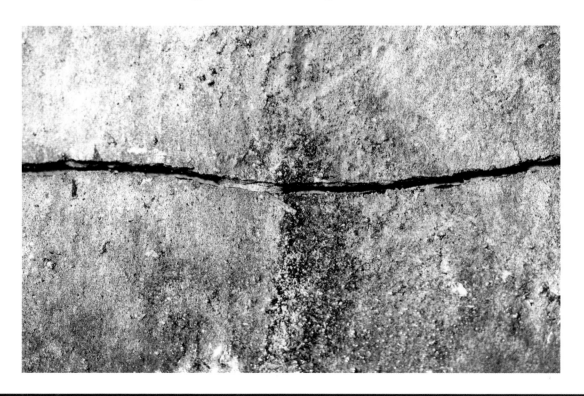

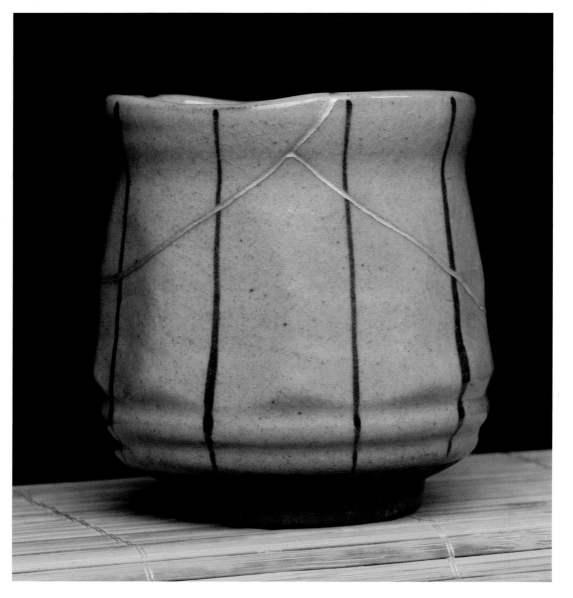

The Zen monk Murata Shuko (1423–1502) is credited with being one of the first practitioners to infuse the philosophy of wabi-sabi into the Japanese tea ceremony. Rather than using the finest implements, he emphasized simple utensils. And while the wealthy and fashionable arranged their ceremonies around clear nights when views of a perfectly full moon were possible, Shuko advised his students to appreciate the half moon, or a partial moon on a cloudy night.

BODY SCAN

Body scan meditation is a kind of mindfulness with razor-sharp focus on the body. Emotions—from anxiety to fear to joy—have physical symptoms. Delight can make us feel lighter, deep sadness can cause tightness in the chest, and stress can be a literal pain in the neck. With a body scan, you take stock of these symptoms and the emotions behind them.

The intent of this meditation is simply to notice, not to judge. In the words of Paul McCartney, let it be.

Time
A thorough body scan can take as long as 45 minutes. If you're pressed for time, you can try a quick 5-minute or 10-minute scan instead.

Posture
Because it can take awhile to complete a body scan, make sure you're comfortable. Most people lie down. Pillows under the knees, neck, or upper back can help reduce pain and keep your body relaxed. If you're worried about falling asleep, you can sit up on a cushion or a chair.

Remember
Your mind will wander, and that's okay. When it does, acknowledge that it has, then gently bring your attention back to the part of your body where you left off.

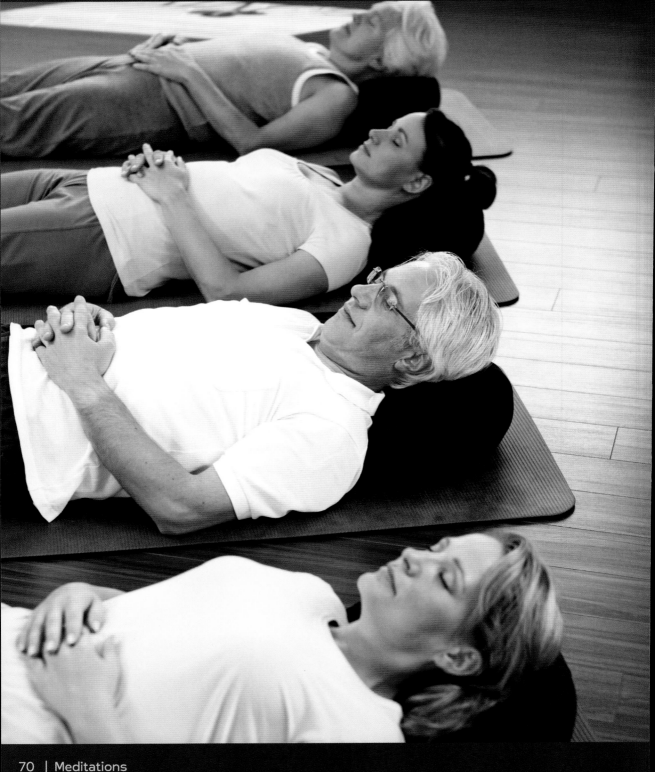

HOW TO DO IT

Step 1
Take a few deep breaths. Breathe in through the nose and out through the mouth.

Step 2
Notice the heaviness of your body. Where does your body come in contact with the floor, bed, or other object beneath you? Feel the pressure at those points.

Step 3
Bring your attention to one toe. Notice every physical sensation you're experiencing with that toe. Is it cold? Warm? Is there pressure or tightness of any kind? What else do you notice?

Step 4
Do the same to the next toe, then the next. When you've gone through all the toes, move on to the soles of your feet, the tops of your feet, your ankles, all the way up to the top of your head.

When you reach a spot that is experiencing tension, breathe into that area. Feel your lungs fill as you inhale, and imagine the oxygen and energy passing through the muscles as you exhale, releasing the tension.

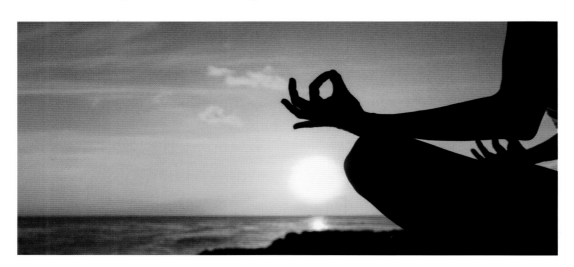

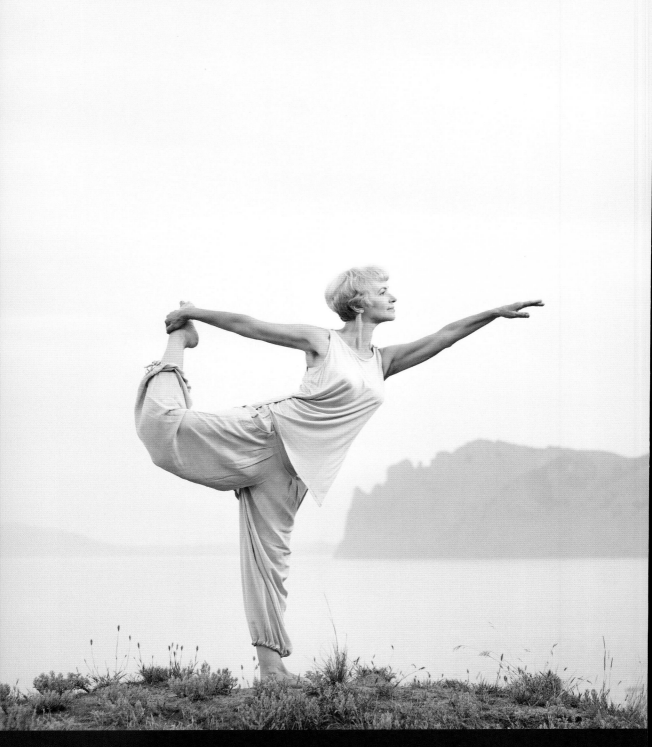

The Brain—is wider than the Sky—
For—put them side by side—
The one the other will contain
With ease—and You—beside—

The Brain is deeper than the sea—
For—hold them—Blue to Blue—
The one the other will absorb—
As Sponges—Buckets—do—

The Brain is just the weight of God—
For—Heft them—Pound for Pound—
And they will differ—if they do—
As Syllable from Sound—

—Emily Dickinson

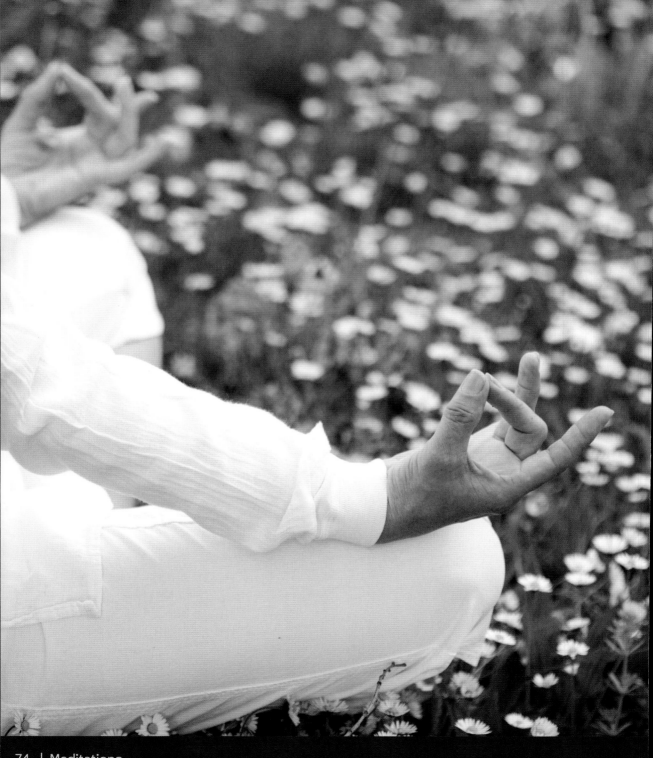

CHAKRA

Chakra is Sanskrit for "wheel." Chakras are believed by some to be the points where the metaphysical self connects to the physical self. The chakras spin, moving energy through the body. When one or more chakras are blocked, others spin faster to compensate. This imbalance then causes difficulties.

Chakra meditation focuses on the seven most important chakras, which are located along the spine and at the top of your head. Some practitioners go through certain body postures, hand positions, and mantras as they meditate. Others—especially beginners—stay simply seated.

Time
Beginners may have sessions lasting 10 to 15 minutes. More seasoned practitioners often meditate for at least 30 minutes.

Posture
Sit in a comfortable position. Legs may be crossed or in a lotus position if you're on the floor or a cushion. If you're sitting in a chair, position yourself so your feet are flat on the floor if you can. Support yourself with cushions behind your back, under your knees, or elsewhere as needed. Keep your back comfortably straight, gaze down or eyes closed.

Remember
Your mind will wander, and that's ok. When it wanders or becomes fixed on a topic, acknowledge that it has. Then gently bring your attention back to your visualization.

HOW TO DO IT

Step 1

Take a few deep breaths. Breathe in through the nose and out through the mouth.

Step 2

Bring your focus to your root chakra, located at the base of your spine. Visualize a ball of energy there, gently glowing red. Imagine your breath flowing into it, making it bigger and brighter.

Step 3

Move to your sacral chakra, just below the navel. Visualize a ball of orange energy. Breathe into it until it matches the size and brightness of your root chakra.

Step 4

Do the same with your solar plexus chakra (which glows yellow), heart (green), throat (blue), third eye (indigo), and finally the crown (violet or white).

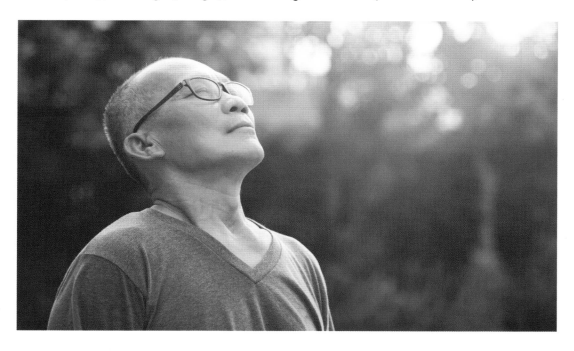

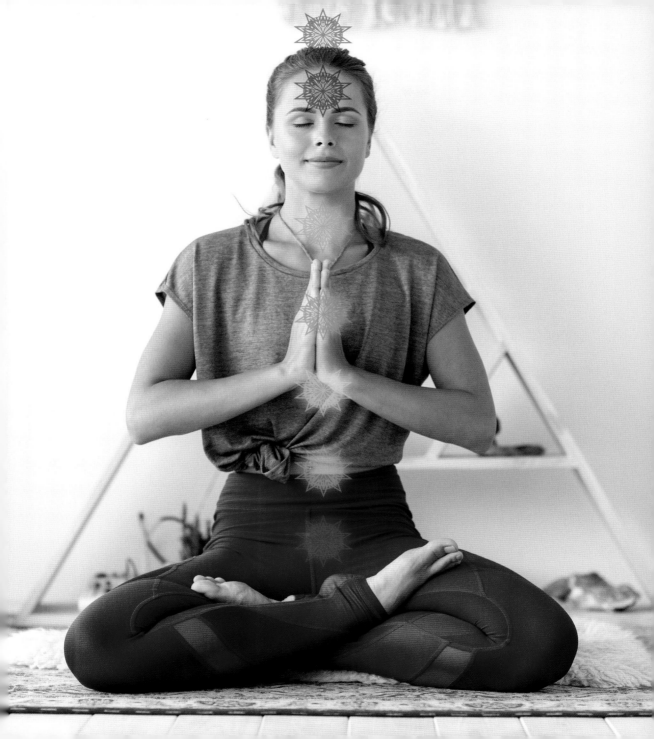

The first chakra is the **root chakra**, located at the base of the spine. Like the strong foundation of a pyramid, the root chakra represents stability and basic sustenance. Its color is red.

The second is the **sacral chakra**, named for its location above the sacrum. The sacrum is the largest vertebra and the one that connects with both sides of your pelvis. This chakra is orange and represents creativity as an integrated part of your mind and energy.

The third, the solar plexus chakra, is found below the sternum. It's named after the radiating cluster of nerves sometimes also called the celiac plexus. This chakra is yellow and associated with both physical digestion and the metaphorical digestion of new ideas.

The fourth, the heart chakra, is associated with circulation, but also with the understanding of the heart as the "emotional brain" of the body. This chakra is green.

The fifth, the throat chakra, is associated with communication and with hormones because of its location among the thyroid, pituitary, and other glands. This chakra is blue.

The sixth, the **third eye chakra**, is the most well-known chakra in the popular imagination. It represents insight, clarity, and intuition or psychic ability. A clear sixth chakra is said to allow you to see your place within the fabric of the universe. This chakra is indigo.

The seventh, the **crown chakra**, is both the top of the head and the upper limit of human existence. This chakra is violet.

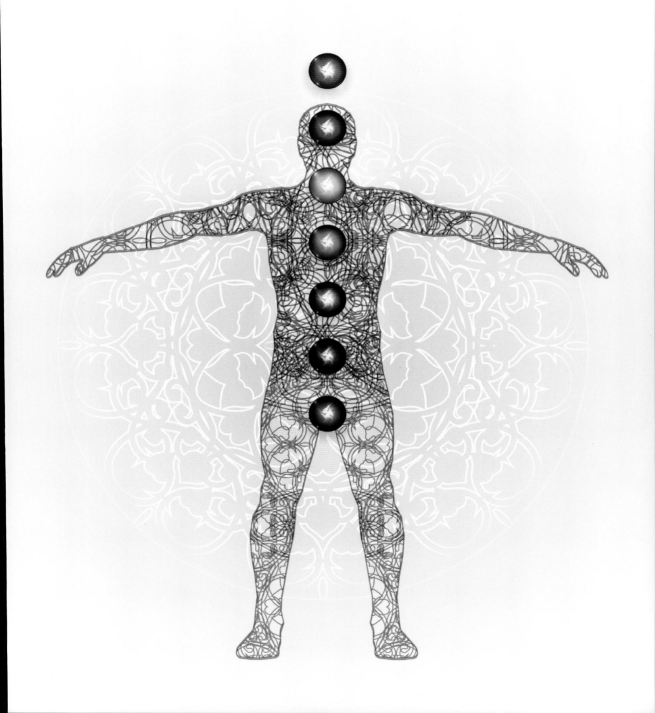

CONTEMPLATIVE READING

Many religions use contemplative reading or similar practices. The goal is to feel a connection to the divine by way of sacred text. In Christian tradition, it's called *Lectio Divina,* or divine reading. It involves spending time with a short section of text and considering it outside of any historical or theological context, creating a deeply personal relationship with the words. The driving question is, roughly, "What is the divine saying to *me, right now.*"

Time
You can spend 10 minutes on the entire process, or 10 or more minutes on each step. Christian monks once practiced by repeating the words six times. A good place to start is with three or four repetitions.

Posture
Make sure you're comfortable, and that you can remain so for the length of your practice.

Remember
Your mind will wander, and that's ok. When it wanders, acknowledge that it has. Then gently bring your attention back to the words. Also, try not to consciously assign a meaning to the passage. Focus instead on how you experience and react to the passage.

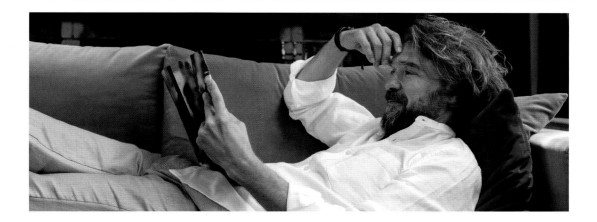

HOW TO DO IT

Step 1
Choose a short section of a sacred text. People often choose something that is one or two sentences long.

Step 2
Read the passage aloud, slowly and deliberately. Listen carefully to the sound of the words. Sit quietly for a few minutes considering what they mean to you.

Step 3
Read the passage aloud again. Try to read it with a different emphasis or rhythm. Sit quietly for a few more minutes.

Step 4
Repeat this process at least once more.

Step 5
Think about how the passage made you feel, any images it sparked in your imagination, and any words or phrases that stuck out to you. Spend several minutes with this process.

Step 6
Focus on a word, phrase, emotion, or vision the passage brought up for you that was very dominant in your mind. Consider what this dominant thought is saying to you, in this moment. Spend several minutes with this process.

Step 7
Let conscious thought fade. Bring your focus to your breath. Breathe naturally.

DANCING MEDITATION

Dancing is as old and as multifaceted as the human species. People dance alone, with a partner, or with a group. There might be strict choreography, a set of steps to be mixed and matched, or something entirely improvised. It can be worship, self-expression, celebration, performance, social interaction, and exercise. It can also be meditation.

Any dance requires a certain amount of mental focus. Your primary attention is usually on your body, while additional attention can be given to the music, a partner, or some choreography. When using dance as a method of meditation, all your attention is on your body and the music, just as you would focus everything on the breath or a mantra in other meditations.

Dance meditation is adaptable to a range of abilities and interests. You can dance across the floor on your feet, swing your arms from a seated position, or just bob your head or tap your toe to the music. The important part is to bring your attention to your movement and how it feels. The music can be anything you want it to be, from hymns, to opera, to EDM. Choose a style of music that naturally speaks to you and, preferably, inspires some positive feeling.

Time
If you're new to dance meditation, try spending 10 to 15 minutes with it at first. That time can be extended to 30 or more minutes as you become more comfortable.

Space
Make sure you have the space needed to move freely. If you'll be on your feet, make sure the floor is clear of obstacles.

Remember
Your mind will wander, and that's ok. When it wanders, acknowledge that it has. Then gently bring your attention back to the music and your movement. Dance freely and without judgement. Dance meditation is not about beauty or skill; it's just about moving.

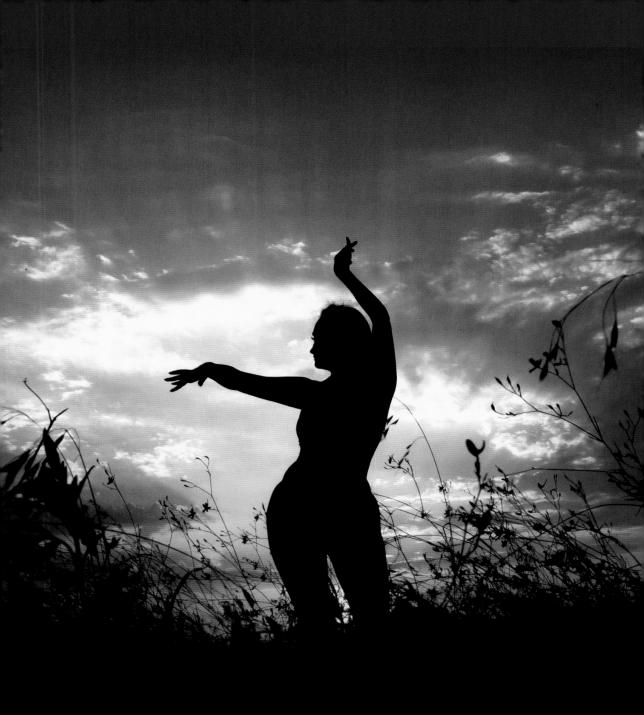

HOW TO DO IT

Step 1

Start the music. Take a few deep breaths to ground yourself. Then return to natural breathing.

Step 2

Bring your focus to the rhythm of the music. Imagine it pulsing within your body. It can help to lightly nod, tap a toe, or tap a finger to the rhythm.

Step 3

Shift your attention to the melody of the music. Notice each note as it passes by.

Step 4

Turn that melody into movement. For example, as the melody goes up, you can raise your arms. As it goes down, you can reach toward the floor. (These are just examples; there's no need for you to follow them.) Move your body by instinct, if you can, without too much thought.

Step 5

Bring your focus to your body as it moves. Note each muscle that drives the movement, and each bone and tendon that supports it.

Step 6

If there is harmony in the music, turn your focus to that. Notice how the harmony interacts with the melody. Incorporate this added complexity to your movement.

I know not what the spirit of a philosopher would like better than to be a good dancer. For the dance is his ideal, and also his art, in the end likewise his sole piety, his "divine service."

—Friedrich Nietzsche

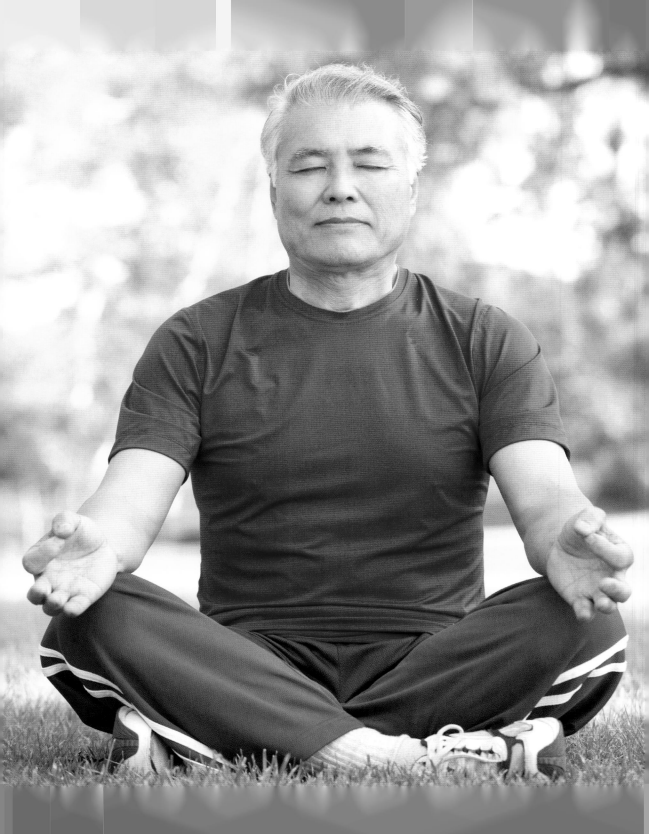

GAZING

This practice is sometimes used in Hatha Yoga, where it's called trataka, but gazing meditation is by no means limited to yogis. It's an excellent method to try if you have trouble keeping your mind focused in other forms of meditation. Gazing meditation involves focusing on a physical object in front of you, such as a candle.

Time
When you first try this meditation, start with 5 to 10 minutes. As you become more comfortable with the practice, you can increase the time.

Posture
Sit in a comfortable position. Legs may be crossed or in a lotus position if you're on the floor or a cushion. If you're sitting in a chair, position yourself so your feet are flat on the floor if you can. Support yourself with cushions behind your back, under your knees, or elsewhere as needed. Keep your back comfortably straight.

Remember
Your mind will wander, and that's ok. When it wanders or becomes fixed on a topic, acknowledge that it has. Then gently bring your attention back to the flame or other object of focus.

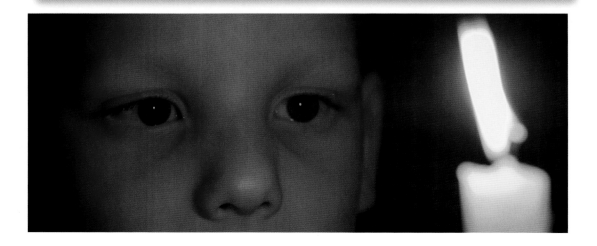

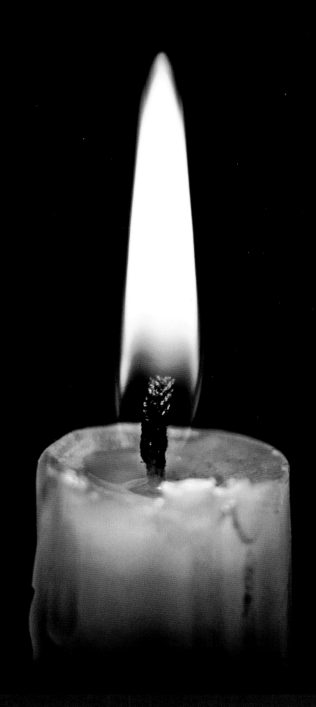

HOW TO DO IT

Step 1
Place a candle on a level surface that is free of anything flammable. The candle should sit a couple of feet from you, at about eye level. Darken the room, if you wish to.

Step 2
Close your eyes and take a few deep breaths. Focus on each inhale and exhale. Then return to natural breathing.

Step 3
Open your eyes and focus on the candle's flame. Try to blink as little as possible. It helps to open your eyes a little wider than usual. If you notice the flame blurring in your vision, consciously bring it back into focus.

Step 4
If the eyes begin to feel strained, close them for a moment to let them rest. You can also cover your eyes with cupped hands. Then return to gazing at the flame.

Step 5
When you are ready, close your eyes and bring the image of the flame up in your mind's eye. Hold it there and concentrate on it, just as you did with your eyes open.

Step 6
If your mind becomes still and the mental image of the flame fades, you can let the image go and remain simply in stillness.

HEARTBEAT

Meditating on your heartbeat brings your focus inward, and it can encourage calmness and clarity. The practice may also help increase empathy.

Some people silently repeat a mantra during this meditation. The mantra is usually one or two syllables so it matches the double beat (ba-dum, ba-dum) of the heart. Kundalini yogis often use Sat Nam ("I am Truth," or "Truth is my essence"). "I am" is another choice.

Time
If you're just beginning with this meditation, start with a goal of 10 minutes. You can increase or decrease the time according to what is comfortable.

Posture
Sit in a comfortable position. Legs may be crossed or in a lotus position if you're on the floor or a cushion. If you're sitting in a chair, position yourself so your feet are flat on the floor if you can. Support yourself with cushions behind your back, under your knees, or elsewhere as needed. Keep your back comfortably straight, gaze down or eyes closed.

Remember
Your mind will wander, and that's ok. When it wanders or becomes fixed on a topic, acknowledge that it has. Then gently bring your attention back to your heartbeat.

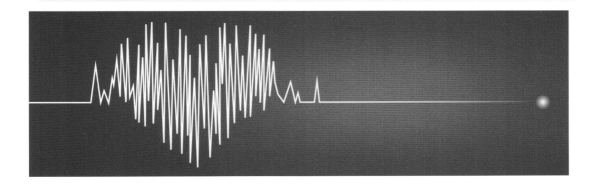

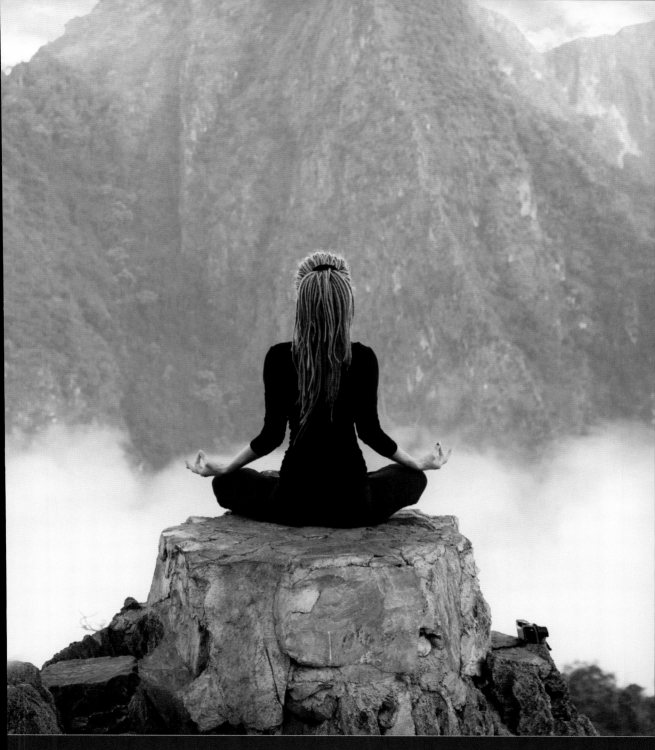

HOW TO DO IT

Step 1
Breathe deeply a few times to ground yourself.

Step 2
Begin to extend your inhales and exhales to perhaps 6 or more seconds each. At the top of your inhale, pause with your breath held. Count to 3, then exhale. Adjust the lengths of your inhale, pause, and exhale if you need to make the breathing pattern comfortable.

Step 3
You should start to notice your heartbeat becoming more obvious, especially when you hold your breath. The longer you hold the breath, the more strongly you'll feel your heartbeat. If you use a mantra, begin repeating it in your mind to the rhythm of your heartbeat.

Step 4
When you're ready, place your fingers on a pulse point. It could be your wrist, throat, temple, or elsewhere. Turn your focus to that beat. Continue repeating any mantra you're using.

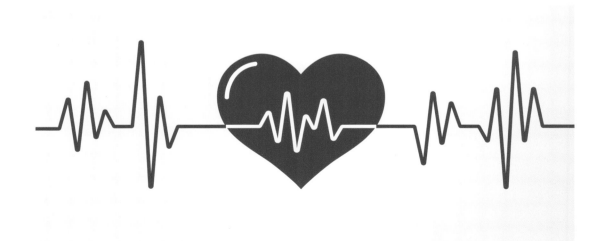

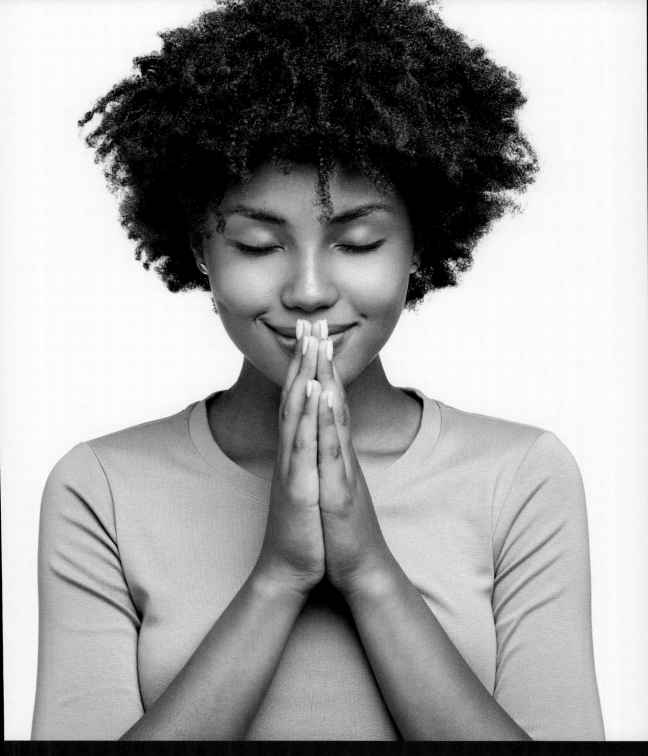

Those who stand on tiptoes

do not stand firmly.

Those who rush ahead

don't get very far.

Those who try to outshine others

dim their own light.

Those who call themselves righteous

can't know how wrong they are.

Those who boast of their accomplishments

diminish the things they have done.

—Lao Tzu

MANTRAS

A mantra is a repeated sound, syllable, word, or phrase that serves as a tool to cultivate focus, intention, or inspiration in the mind. It is usually spoken or thought over and over again in a steady rhythm. The word mantra is often associated specifically with Hinduism and Buddhism, though other religions also make use of repeated words, and many people have adopted mantras into non-religious meditations.

Mantras can be part of a meditation practice in a huge variety of ways. You can chant them aloud or repeat them in your head. They can be short or long, religious or secular, in any language, or in no language at all. You can add them to any part of your meditation, or just use them at stressful moments in your day. You can repeat your mantra a certain number of times, for a specific length of time, or simply until you're ready to move on. It's all up to you. All a mantra needs to do is help you stay true to the intention of your practice.

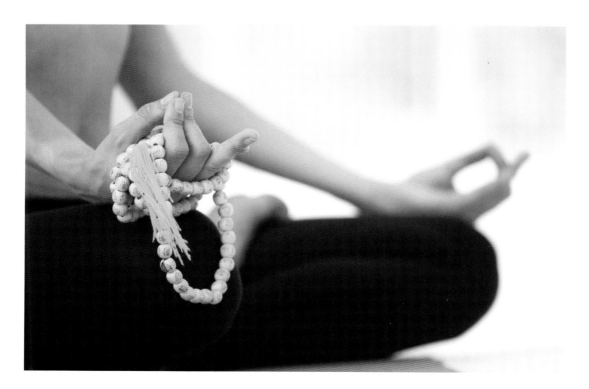

OM

You're likely familiar with Om. The syllable is synonymous with meditation, and it is sacred in Hinduism, Buddhism, and other religions. Scriptures connect it to creation and the divine, and describe it as the origin of all sounds. Many practitioners see Om as the tool that sends the spirit to enlightenment or the divine. Picture a bow, arrow, and target. The bow is Om, the arrow is the spirit, the target is the divine.

Om is pronounced with three sounds: AH-OO-MM (this is why you can sometimes find it spelled "AUM"). The three parts can represent a variety of trinities, including past, present, and future; creation, preservation, and liberation; the physical plane, mental plane, and deep-sleep state; and goodness, passion, and darkness. A fourth—and equally important—part of the syllable is the silence that comes at the end of it.

Time
Some people (yogis, for example) chant Om a few times at the beginning or end of a practice. Others chant for perhaps 45 minutes or more. Many Buddhists chant a mantra a certain number of times, keeping count on a string of beads such as a mala.

Posture
Sit in a comfortable position. Legs may be crossed or in a lotus position if you're on the floor or a cushion. If you're sitting in a chair, position yourself so your feet are flat on the floor if you can. Support yourself with cushions behind your back, under your knees, or elsewhere as needed. Keep your back comfortably straight, gaze down or eyes closed.

Remember
Your mind will wander, and that's ok. That's part of what you're working on with this meditation. When it wanders or becomes fixed on a topic, acknowledge that it has. Then gently bring your attention back to your meditation.

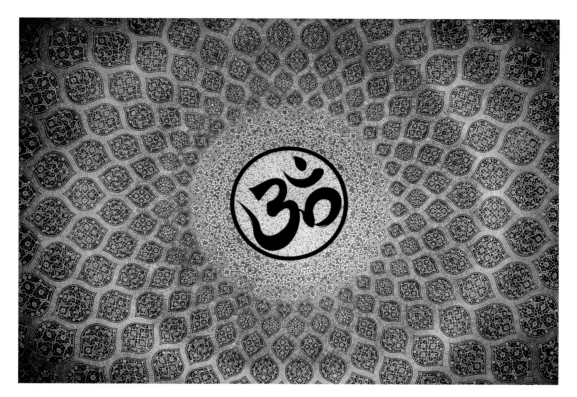

HOW TO DO IT

Breathe naturally. Say or think "Om" during an exhale. The length of your Om should match the time it takes to complete the exhale. Transition smoothly between each of Om's three sounds, spending a few seconds on each. You can repeat Om with every exhale, or you can take breaths in between each repetition.

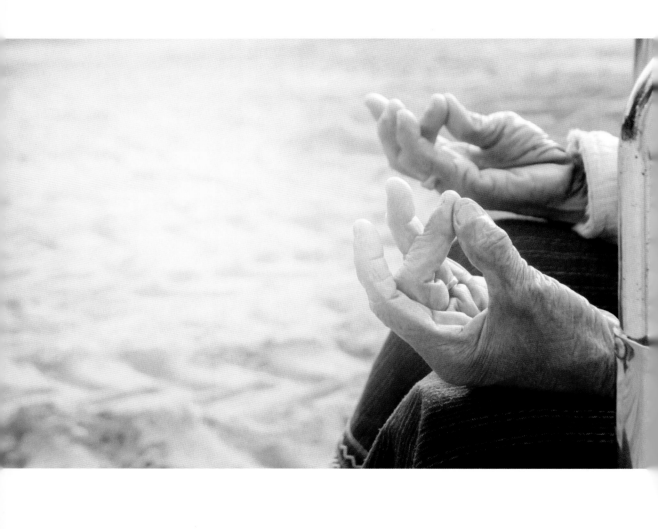

I AM

A mantra like "I am" is a very straightforward, personal method of meditation. The phrase can be said in any language, though it often resonates strongest when it is in your first language.

"I am" has a particular connection to certain religions. In Sanskrit, the phrase is "So Hum," or literally "I am that/he." In Vedic philosophies, So Hum represents the connection between the individual and the universe, with "I am" being the personal and "that" the universal. In meditating, many practitioners combine this with Om, for "Om So Hum."

This phrase is also important in Judaism, Christianity, and Islam. According to sacred texts, God described himself to the prophet Moses as, "I am that I am." In Hebrew, this is "Ehyeh Asher Ehyeh," but anyone wishing to use it in their meditation can of course repeat the phrase in English, Spanish, or whatever language resonates most.

The mantra doesn't need to be religious. Repeating "I am" is an excellent way to include self-exploration and self-reflection in a secular meditation practice.

Time
A good place to start is 10 to 15 minutes. As you become more comfortable and familiar with the practice, you can increase the time to 30 minutes, 45 minutes, or more.

Posture
Sit in a comfortable position. Legs may be crossed or in a lotus position if you're on the floor or a cushion. If you're sitting in a chair, position yourself so your feet are flat on the floor if you can. Support yourself with cushions behind your back, under your knees, or elsewhere as needed. Keep your back comfortably straight, gaze down or eyes closed.

Remember
Your mind will wander, and that's ok. When it wanders or becomes fixed on a topic, acknowledge that it has. Then gently bring your attention back to the sound and meaning of the mantra.

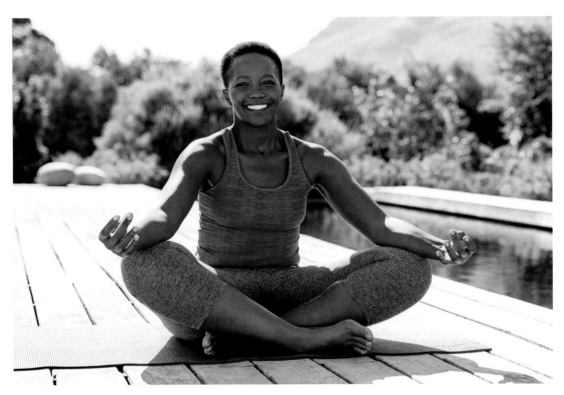

HOW TO DO IT

As with an Om meditation, breathe naturally. Let the rhythm of your mantra match the rhythm of your breath. For example, as you inhale, slowly go through the first part of the mantra, "I." As you exhale, go through the second part, "Am."

POSITIVE AFFIRMATIONS

Positive affirmations are helpful, loving thoughts. In essence, positive affirmations are sentences or phrases that describe something you love about yourself, hope for, or are working toward.

Time

You can spend 5 or 10 minutes with positive affirmations at the beginning or end of a meditation session, or you can focus on them for an entire session. You might also pull these out for a quick 30 seconds when you experience stress or just needa pick-me-up.

Posture

If you're sitting, find a comfortable position. Legs may be crossed or in a lotus position if you're on the floor or a cushion. If you're sitting in a chair, position yourself so your feet are flat on the floor if you can. Support yourself with cushions behind your back, under your knees, or elsewhere as needed. Keep your back comfortably straight, gaze down or eyes closed. If you're on the move and just taking a moment for this exercise, you can be in any posture that suits the situation.

Remember

Your mind will wander, and that's ok. When it wanders or becomes fixed on a topic, acknowledge that it has. Then gently bring your attention back to the sound and meaning of your affirmations.

HOW TO CREATE AFFIRMATIONS

Step 1

What is something you value about yourself or your life? Are you strong? Curious? Are there people around you whom you love? Do you enjoy singing, writing, shooting hoops? Turn your choice into a sentence stating that you recognize and appreciate it, such as "I appreciate that I am strong."

Step 2

What is a state of mind you wish to cultivate? Bravery? Calmness? Compassion? Use your choice in a sentence with "I am," such as "I am brave."

Step 3

How do you want to feel about yourself or the world around you, or what is something you know to be true but often lose sight of? These can be harder to pinpoint. Examples include, "I am worthy," "I love myself," and "My emotions are valid."

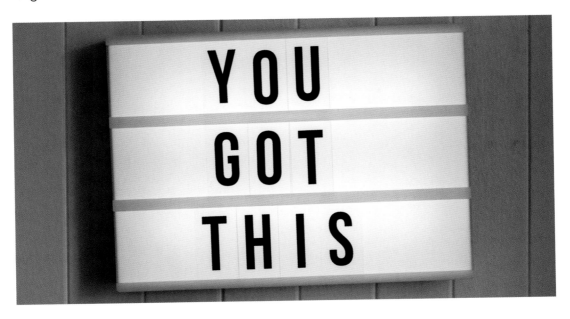

OTHER MANTRAS

There are countless other mantras to create or adopt. What are sounds, words, or phrases that grant you comfort, help you ground yourself, or inspire you? Below are a few categories of mantras that have helped other people.

Prayers

Prayers are a form of religious meditation. Many religions have blessings, litanies, statements of praise or thanks, and other ritual words. Prayers may also be a single divine name or long quotes of scripture. Examples include Catholic rosary prayers and dhikr in Sufism.

Poems and Songs

By design, poems and songs condense complex thoughts, emotions, and experiences into a series of well-chosen words. As a result, these writings are fertile ground for mantras. Whether you use a fragment of a song or the whole of an epic poem, meditating on these words can remind you of your intention, focus your mind, and reveal new layers of meaning in the words themselves.

Famous Quotes

Have you ever run across a quote from a book, a speech, a film, or any other medium, that inspired or calmed you? These words can be useful as mantras as well, as you repeat them and reflect on their meaning.

Sounds

A particular sound can help you focus or calm your mind. A basic mm or ng hum is an example. These are best done aloud so you can feel the vibration in your face, jaw, throat, or chest. It also acts as a tool to become conscious of your breathing. Repeating a melody or rhythm (simple or complex) is another method.

Time

As with other mantra meditations, the time you spend with any of these mantras depends on your intention. You may just need a brief moment before walking out the door to work. You can also chant for much longer, setting a timer or keeping track of repetitions on a string of beads.

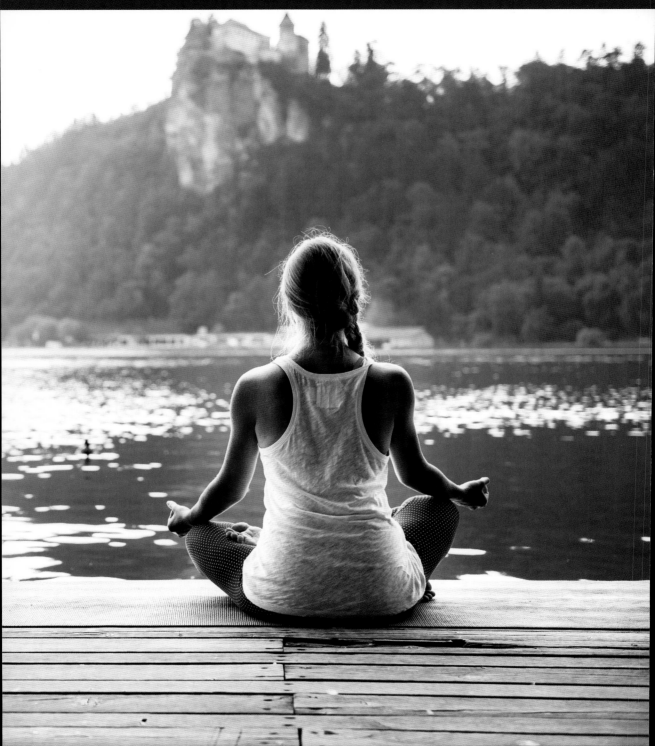

Meditate on the sound of OM, knowing that therein lies the Lord of Love. May His blessing take you out of darkness.

—The Mundaka Upanishad

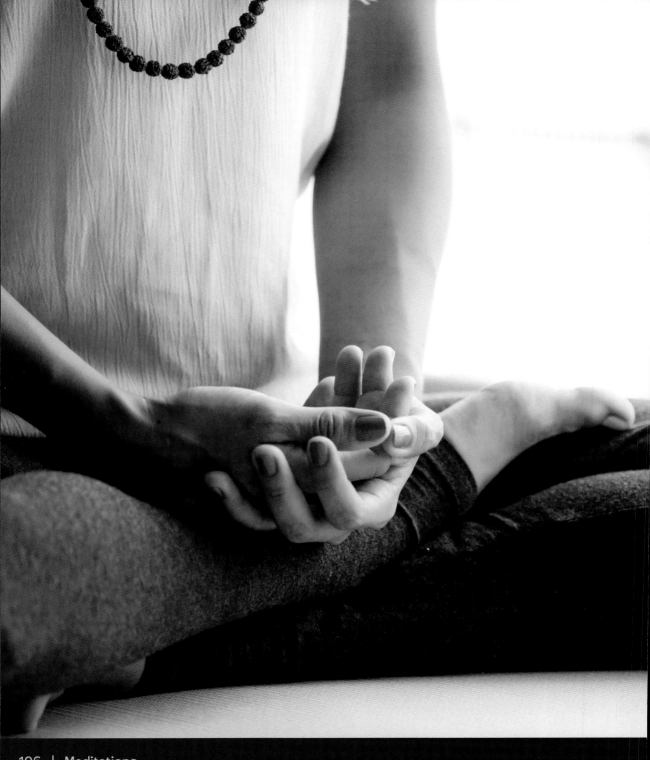

METTA MEDITATION

If you want to put more love and compassion into the world, Metta meditation is a wonderful way to do it. Metta is a word for a kind and friendly love in the Pali language. For this reason, English speakers often call the practice loving-kindness meditation.

Metta is a central concept in Buddhism. It is one of the four essential mental states that together can lead to enlightenment. (The other three are compassion, joy for others, and equanimity.) As such, many Buddhists include Metta meditation in their religious practice.

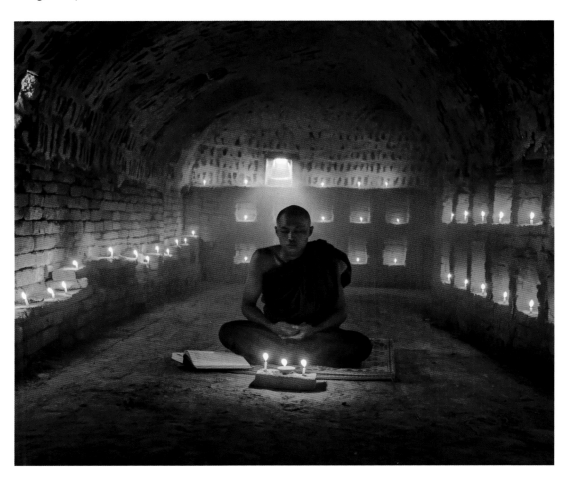

Time

This meditation can take as long as you need it to. Beginners may start by spending 10 or 20 minutes meditating. Those who are more practiced can spend 45 minutes or more with it.

Metta meditation is done in stages, beginning with yourself and expanding outwards. If you're a beginner, take it slow. You can do the meditation in pieces, completing only the first stage or two in a session. Add stages to your practice when you're ready. Alternatively, you can complete all of the stages in one session, spending a short period on each stage and expanding that time as you become more comfortable.

Posture

Sit in a comfortable position. Legs may be crossed or in a lotus position if you're on the floor or a cushion. If you're sitting in a chair, position yourself so your feet are flat on the floor if you can. Support yourself with cushions behind your back, under your knees, or elsewhere as needed. Keep your back comfortably straight, gaze down or eyes closed.

Remember

Your mind will wander, and that's okay. When it does, acknowledge that it has, then gently bring your attention back to the light of loving-kindness and, if you are repeating a mantra, to the words and meaning of that mantra.

If the practice seems mechanical or insincere at first, keep with it. Change may be happening even if you don't immediately notice it.

HOW TO DO IT

Metta meditation is done in stages. Visualization is a big part of it, and many people repeat mantras as well.

Your mantra can be any phrase or phrases that are positive and loving, such as "May I feel happiness and peace," or "May I be safe and healthy." You can say the mantra out loud or in your head.

Stage 1

Begin with yourself. Imagine loving-kindness as a light that comes from and surrounds you. Feel the warmth of it. Repeat your mantra in the first person, as in, "May I be safe and healthy."

Stage 2

When you're ready, think of a person in your life whom you like. Hold that person and all the things you love about them in your mind. Imagine your light of loving-kindness surrounding your loved one. Repeat your mantra again, turning it toward the person, as in, "May you be safe and healthy."

Stage 3

Think of a person toward whom you feel neutral. This is someone you do not particularly like or dislike. Perhaps the person is an acquaintance or a stranger. In your mind's eye, see the light of loving-kindness around this person. Repeat your mantra, applying its meaning to them, too.

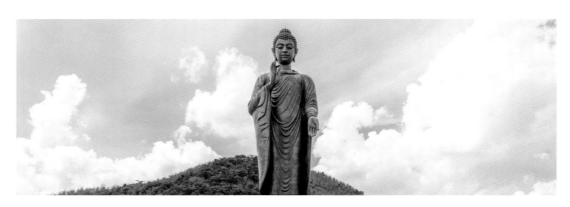

Stage 4

Think of a person you do not like, or with whom you have difficulty. Be gentle with yourself if ill feelings bubble up in your mind as you think of the person. Acknowledge the feelings and let them go, reminding yourself of the person's humanity. Think of them positively. Again, surround them in the light of your loving-kindness and repeat your mantra.

Stage 5

Imagine all these people—yourself, the loved one, the neutral person, and the disliked person—together in a close group. Imagine the light of loving-kindness filling and surrounding all of you at once. Repeat your mantra for the entire group, as in, "May we feel happiness and peace."

Stage 6

In your mind's eye, extend that light out to include the people immediately around you. Expand it to include your neighborhood, then your town, your country, and your continent. Keep going until the light encompasses the entire world.

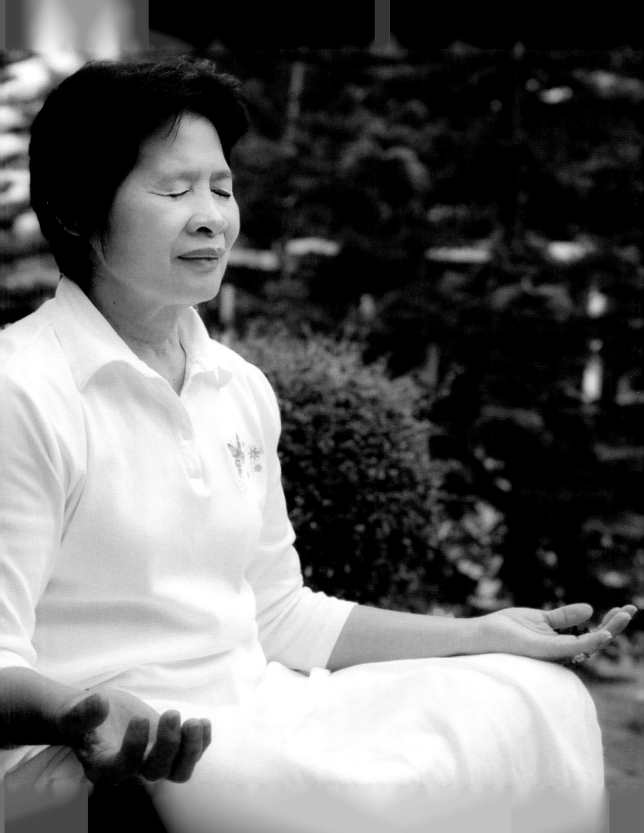

MINDFULNESS

We spend a lot of time stuck in the past or the future. Whether negative (regretting something said the night before) or positive (daydreaming about an upcoming dinner date), these thoughts pull us away from the here and now. This can increase stress and wreak havoc on our ability to focus.

Mindfulness meditation is an effort to hit the brakes on runaway thoughts by focusing on one single, natural thing: the breath. The practice is less about clearing the mind, and more about becoming aware of it. This process grounds us securely in the present moment. Practitioners report calmer minds, more regenerative relaxation, and overall less stress.

Time
It's better to practice this meditation in short sessions several times a week, rather than in one or two long sessions. With this in mind, a session may be as short as 3 to 5 minutes, especially if you're just starting out. With time and practice, you'll become more comfortable with sessions lasting 45 minutes or more.

Posture
Sit in a comfortable position. Legs may be crossed or in a lotus position if you're on the floor or a cushion. If you're sitting in a chair, position yourself so your feet are flat on the floor if you can. Support yourself with cushions behind your back, under your knees, or elsewhere as needed. Keep your back comfortably straight, gaze down or eyes closed.

Remember
Your mind will wander, and that's ok. When it wanders or becomes fixed on a topic, acknowledge that it has. Then gently bring your attention back to your breath.

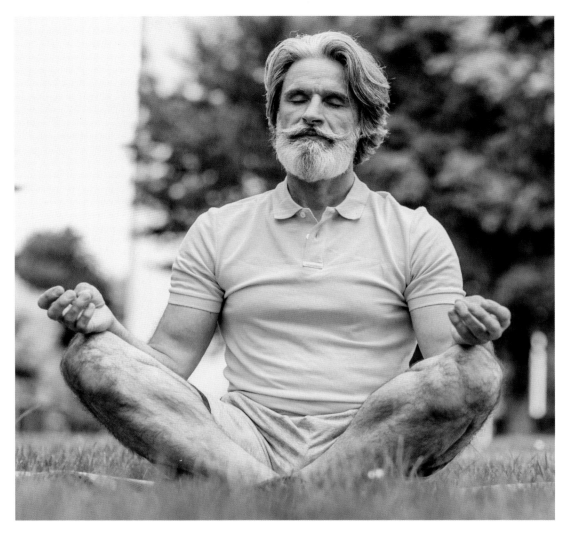

Mindfulness is not zoning out, or avoiding reality and our problems. Mindfulness is facing the realities of life and staying fully present to the solutions that are all around us. Mindfulness is paying attention, because it is only in the present moment that we experience synchronicities and miracles. Only in the present moment are we truly in rhythm with the heartbeat of life as it is, and not as we want it to be. It is there we find our answers

HOW TO DO IT

Step 1
Take a few deep breaths. Breathe in through the nose and out through the mouth.

Step 2
Return to your natural breath, and gently bring your attention to it. Don't change or control your breathing, just be aware of it. Consider the physical sensation of the air moving into your body, filling your lungs, and then moving out.

Step 3 (optional)
If it helps, you can count each inhale and exhale (inhale 1, exhale 2, inhale 3, and so on). Continue until you reach six, then start again from one.

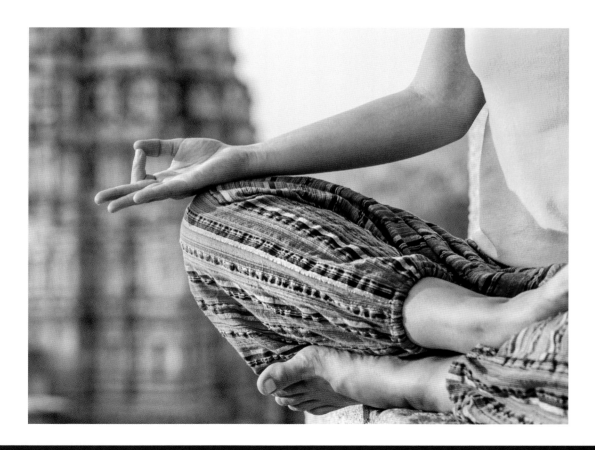

EVERY DAY

One way to practice mindfulness throughout the day is by pausing before taking an action. So before you head into the office, take a few minutes to quietly sit at your desk or in your car before tackling the tasks of the day. Take a few deep breaths, take note of the sights and sounds nearby, and allow your thoughts and feelings to come and go. You can also pause in other areas of the day—before answering a ringing phone, for example, or before heading into a meeting. Simply take a quick deep breath, or pause to collect your thoughts and focus on your feelings. You can take a few moments before answering emails, as well. Read through each message and then take some time before forming responses. How does each message make you feel? Stressed? Overwhelmed? Appreciated? Undervalued? Whatever emotion is conjured up, accept it without judgment and then continue. This may even help you to approach messages in a less emotional, more professional way throughout the day.

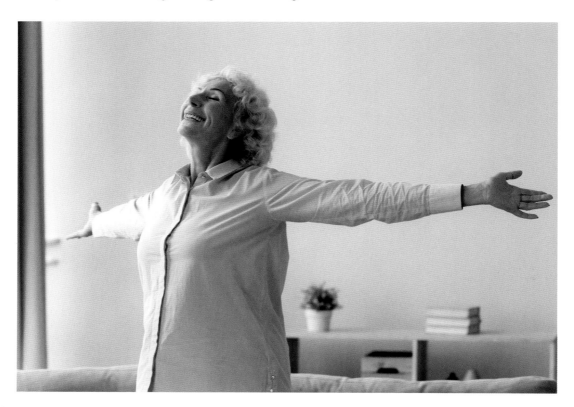

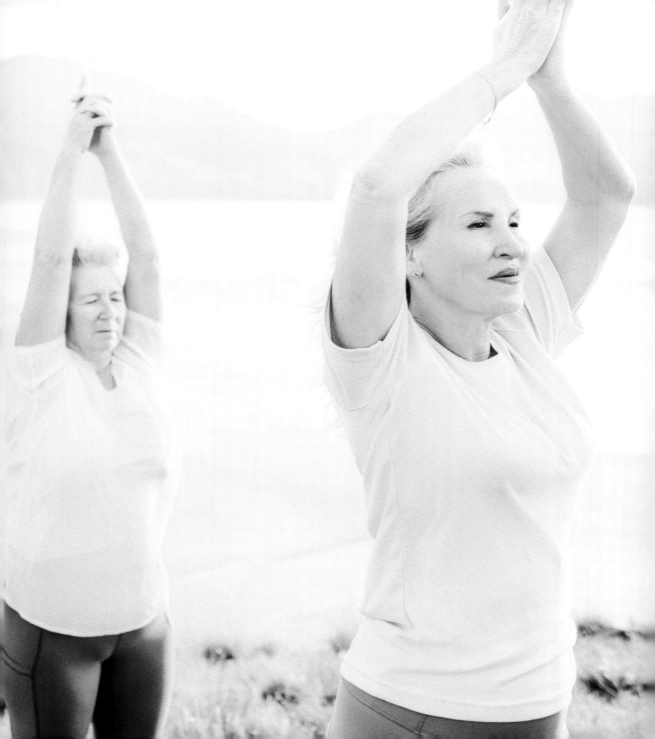

Fear less, hope more; eat less, chew more; whine less, breathe more; hate less, love more; and all good things are yours.

—a Swedish proverb

NOTING

The process of noting is a tool to help you stay present in the moment. It's particularly useful for people who struggle with a wandering, preoccupied mind. In noting, you notice and label each thought, emotion, or physical sensation distracting you with a simple, single word. Every label is neutral, without judgement or any attempt to change or control.

In the short term, noting gives a wandering mind something relatively active to do, which helps you stay focused and mindful as you meditate. Noting can also help you recognize the thoughts, emotions, or physical sensations that are most heavily on your mind. In the long term, you can learn patterns in your thoughts and feelings. When the time is right, you can then respond to the patterns. This kind of awareness can also help you resist obsessive thinking or preoccupation.

There are a few different types of labeling you can use in your practice.
- Very basic, general labels, such as "this," or "here"
- More specific labels, such as "warmth," "wanting," "excitement," or "tingling"
- Labels describing the type of sensation being experienced, such as, "seeing," "hearing," "feeling," or "thinking"
- Naming the parts of the breath, such as "rising" with an inhale, and "falling" with an exhale

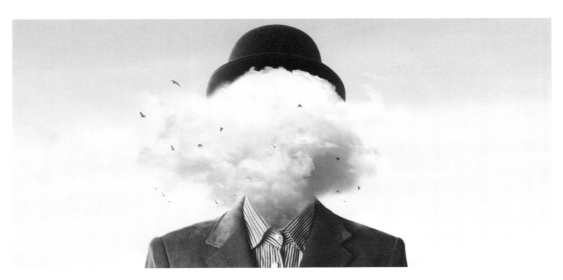

Time
Generally speaking, you can use a noting technique when and however long you need to. It can last 20 minutes and help you enter a mindful state at the beginning of a meditation session. Or you can use the technique for a few moments, breaths, or minutes when you mind becomes particularly distracted from your meditation.

Posture
Use a posture that matches the main meditation method you're using, whether its seated Vipassana, a prone body scan, or a body position in yoga.

Remember
If noting starts to feel mechanical, take a brief break from it. You can come back to it in a few minutes, or if you need, in a few days. There is no "right" or "wrong" label. Use whatever word comes to mind. You don't have to note everything. Note experiences that are dominating your attention. It's okay if the same label comes up over and over again. When it does, note each occurrence until the experience fades or is replaced by another thought.

HOW TO DO IT

Step 1
When a thought, emotion, or physical sensation starts to predominate your focus, take a moment to give it a label. Think it silently in your mind. Then move on from it.

Step 2
Your mind may calm and quieten as you meditate. Let your labels follow, becoming quieter and more nebulous. For example, you may find yourself going from "coolness," to "this," to "hmm."

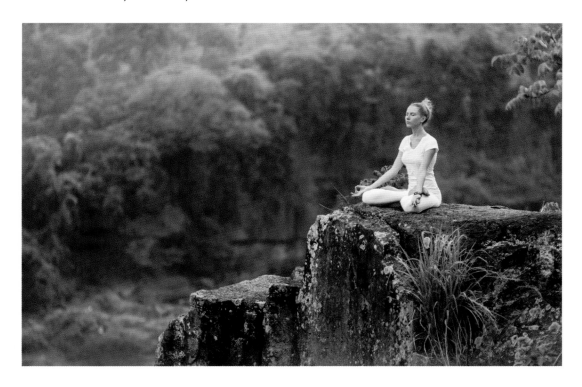

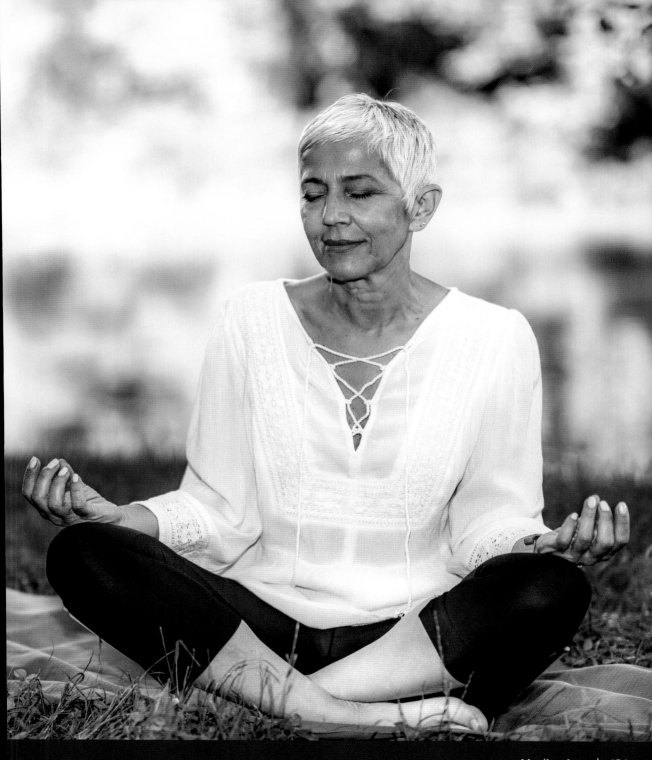

PROGRESSIVE MUSCLE RELAXATION

Progressive muscle relaxation is a technique many people use to combat stress, anxiety, insomnia, digestive issues, high blood pressure, cancer pain, headaches, and a lot of other issues. Basically, you go through your body one muscle group at a time, tensing and releasing each group. The process helps the muscles relax and, as your body relaxes, your mind follows. Some people begin the process with their hands, moving up to the forehead then down to the feet. Others move from the feet to the head.

Time
A full run-through takes about 10 to 20 minutes. Try this technique without setting a timer, though, and focus more on how your body feels rather than how much time has passed.

Posture
Most people lie down for the duration of this exercise, especially when they're using it to help them fall asleep. You can also sit up on a chair or other support. Just make sure you're comfortable and have a little space to move around.

Remember
Your mind will wander, and that's ok. When it wanders, acknowledge that it has. Then gently bring your attention back to the sound. Tense your muscles hard, but not so hard that you feel pain. You can tense and release a muscle group more than once, until you feel your muscles truly relaxing. You can also go through your entire body, then start over again.

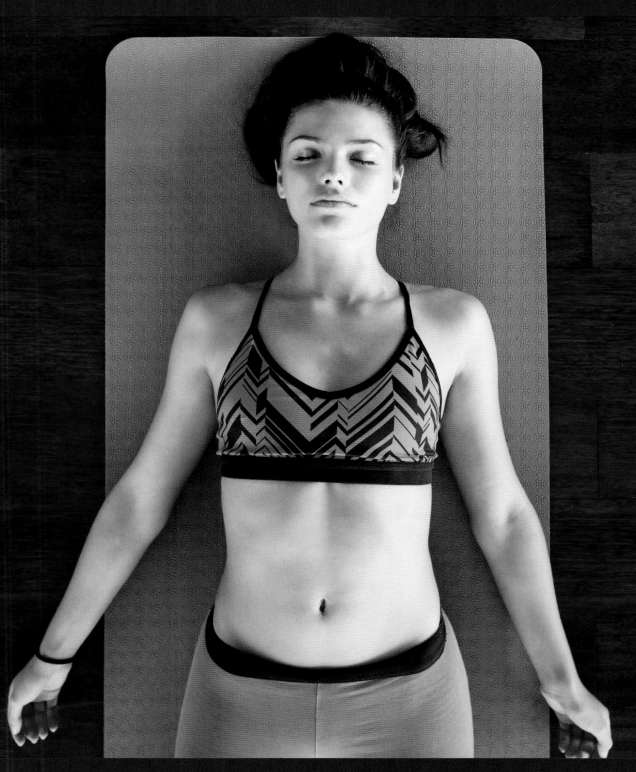

Step 1

As you inhale, tense your hands by making fists. Stay here for 5 to 10 seconds.

Step 2

Exhale slowly, completely releasing the tension.

Step 3

Take about 30 seconds to take stock of any physical changes in your hands and forearms. How do the muscles feel?

Step 4

Inhale, bringing your hands to your shoulders and tensing your biceps. Stay here for 5 to 10 seconds. Then exhale and release the tension. Notice any changes in your upper arms.

Step 5

Continue down through each muscle group.
Shoulders: Shrug, holding the shoulders up around your ears.
Forehead: Raise your eyebrows as high as you can.
Eyes and cheeks: Squeeze your eyes shut.
Jaw: Smile as widely as possible.
Lips: Tightly purse your lips.
Back of the neck: Press the back of the head into the floor, or place a hand on the back of your head and use your neck muscles to press against the hand.

Step 5 (cont.)

Front of the neck: Place a hand on your forehead and use your neck muscles to press into the hand.

Upper back: Roll your shoulders back to press your shoulder blades together, pushing your chest out.

Chest: Breathe in and hold your breath for a moment.

Stomach: Suck your belly in tightly.

Hips and buttocks: Squeeze your buttock muscles together.

Thighs: Clench your thigh muscles.

Calves: Curl your toes back.

Feet: Point your toes away from you, curling the foot.

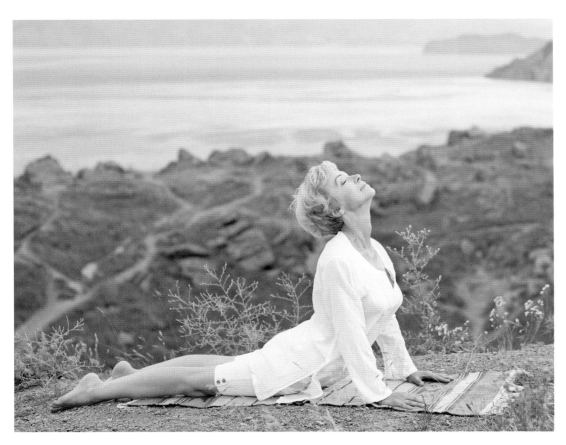

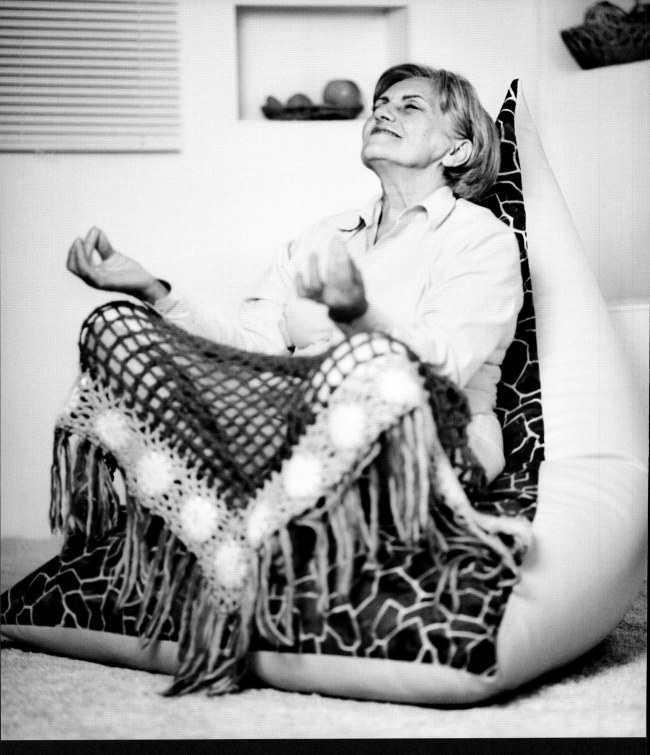

All that we are is the result of what we have thought: It is founded on our thoughts, it is made up of our thoughts. If a man speaks or acts with a pure thought, happiness follows him, like a shadow that never leaves him.

—the Dhammapada

QIGONG

Qigong first developed thousands of years ago in China. Its careful combination of movement, breath, and focused intention is designed to open up and control the body's flow of qi, which can be roughly defined as breath or life energy. Practitioners who've harnessed their qi can use it in healing, in martial arts, or as a spiritual path. Different movements can also affect the body differently: some movements calm, while others invigorate.

Qigong is generally performed by repeating one cyclical movement several times before moving on to the next. As you practice, move gradually, feeling the energy within each moment. Breathe deeply from the belly. Pay attention to how each inhale and exhale fits into the movement. And feel free to adapt the movements as you need to so they suit your body.

Most people—especially beginners—attend classes in Qigong. This way, they have an experienced expert correcting their movements. There's also often a sense of community among classmates.

There are many movements in Qigong. A few are in the next pages.

Time
Qigong classes tend to be around an hour long. If you want to just dip your toes into the practice before attending a class, try spending 10 to 15 minutes with the movements.

Posture
Make sure you have plenty of space needed to move your limbs freely.

Remember
Your mind will wander, and that's ok. When it wanders, acknowledge that it has. Then gently bring your attention back to the breath and your movement.

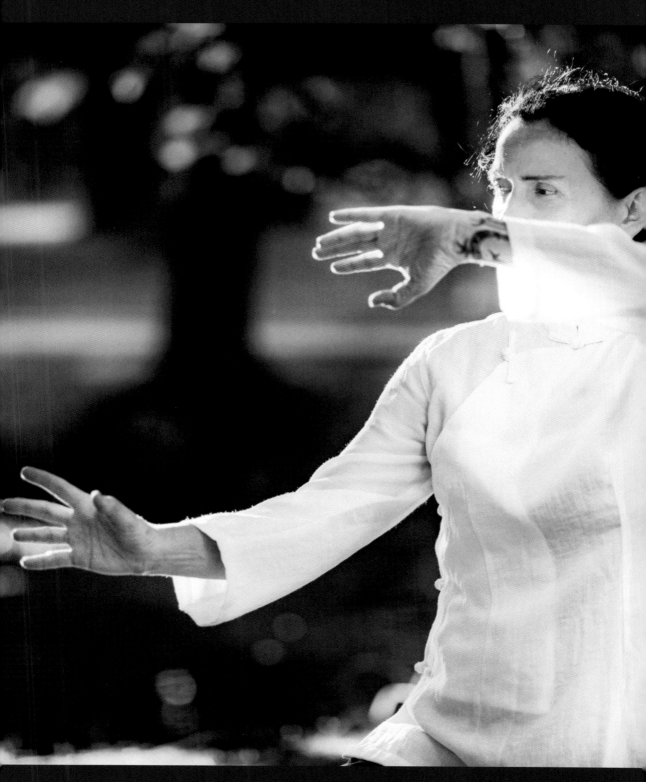

RAISING ARMS

Step 1
Begin in a relaxed but upright standing posture. Feet are hip-width apart, toes pointing forward. Let your arms hang at your sides, palms facing in. Your gaze should be relaxed and unfocused.

Step 2
As you exhale slowly, bend your knees slightly to sink down a little. Rotate your wrists so your palms face to the back.

Step 3
Inhale slowly, straightening your legs to rise back up. Lift your arms in front of you to about shoulder height. Keep your elbows and wrists slightly bent, your fingers relaxed, and palms facing down.

Step 4
Exhale, lowering your arms to your sides and bending your knees.

Step 5
Repeat the cycle of raising with an inhale and lowering with an exhale.

Step 6
When you're ready to end the movement, return to your standing posture in step 1.

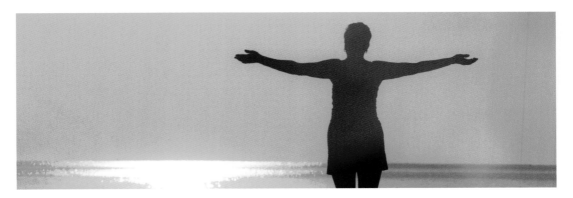

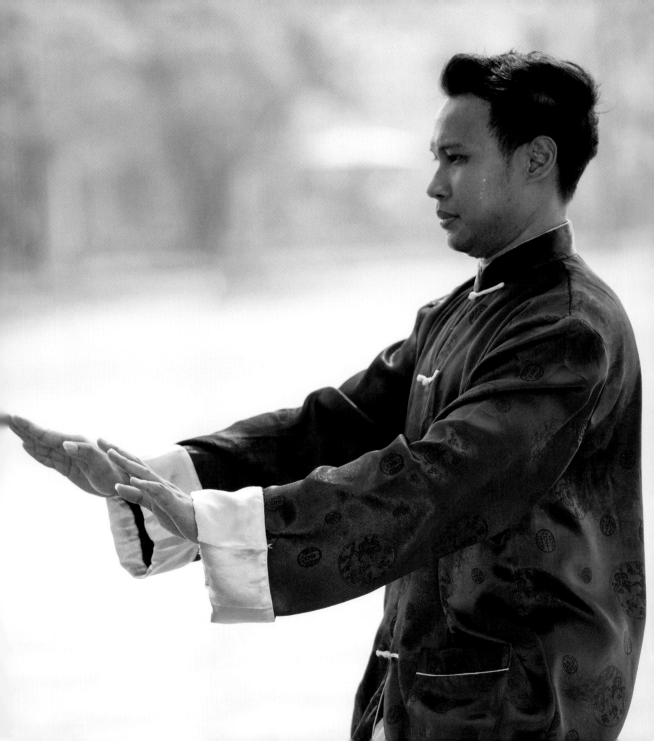

CLOUD HANDS

Step 1
Begin in a relaxed but upright standing posture. Feet are hip-width apart, toes pointing forward. Let your arms hang at your sides, palms facing in. Your gaze should be relaxed and unfocused.

Step 2
Shift your weight to your right leg. Bend the right knee a little as you do so.

Step 3
Extend the left leg out to the side. Gently set the left foot down a few inches from its starting position.

Step 4
Shift your weight to the center, between your feet, and straighten your legs.

Step 5
Lift your left arm, elbow bent, so the elbow points left and your forearm reaches in front of you. Your palm is in front of the center of your chest, facing down.

Step 6
Lift your right arm to waist height, rounded but not fully bent at the elbow. Reach it out in front of you, palm facing left.

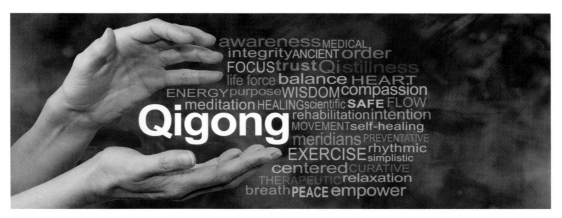

Step 7

Inhale and transfer your weight to the left leg, bending your left knee a little as you do so. Allow your arms to flow to the left as you move, left arm straightening and right elbow bending.

Step 8

Shift your arms so the left is straightened at waist height, right is bent at chest height.

Step 9

Exhale as you shift your weight to the center, then inhale and continue to the right.

Step 10

Switch your arms again (right straight at waist, left bent at chest). Exhale as you shift your weight to the center, inhale as you continue to the left.

Step 11

Continue swaying from left to right, moving your arms in graceful circles. When you're done, return to your standing posture.

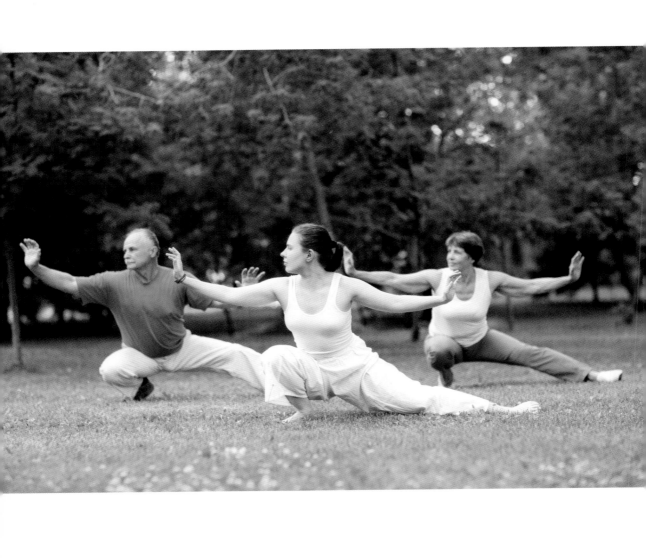

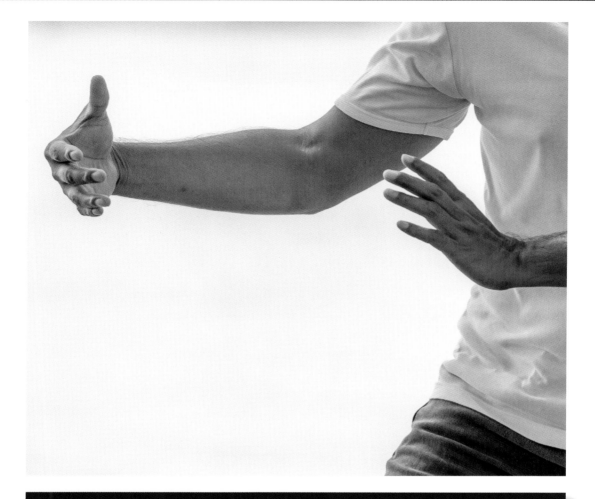

Tai Chi

Tai Chi, sometimes called Taijiquan or Tai Chi Chuan, is closely related to Qigong. The major differences between the two lay in their complexity, approaches to movement, and application. Tai Chi practice consists of sequences of movements, rather than Qigong's usual repetition of single movements, and this means Tai Chi can take a lot longer to learn. Technique is also more rigid in Tai Chi. As for application, Tai Chi is considered a martial art. Qigong is usually more of a wellness-focused practice. That said, Qigong movements and philosophies are often used in Tai Chi, and many people today use Tai Chi purely as a method of meditation or exercise, rather than a martial art.

If you want to become whole,

first let yourself become broken.

If you want to become straight,

first let yourself become twisted.

If you want to become full,

first let yourself become empty.

If you want to become new,

first let yourself become old.

Those whose desires are few get them,

those whose desires are great go astray.

—Lao Tzu

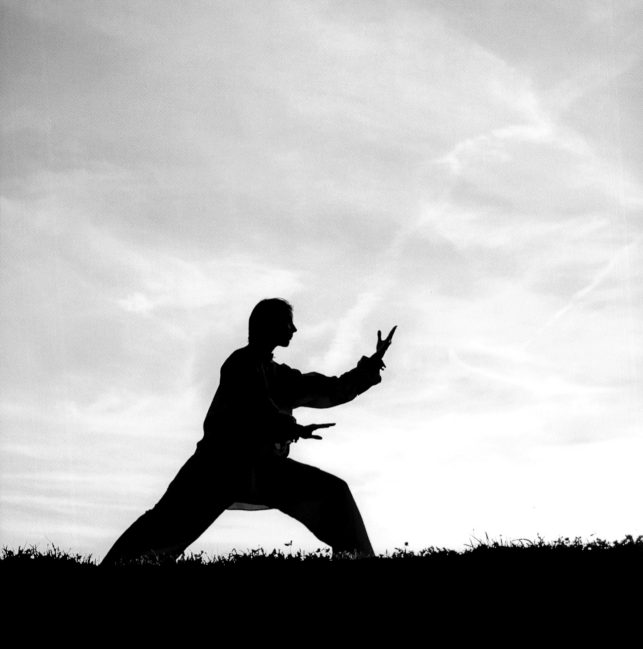

SELF REFLECTION

While most meditations involve letting thoughts and emotions go, a more reflective method is sometimes useful. Self-reflection meditation is a conscious and deliberate effort to study and understand yourself. You can use it to regularly check in on any changes or shifts in your life or identity that have taken place. It can also be a handy tool to work through a feeling or memory that preoccupies you.

Time
Some people practice self-reflection once a week or once a month. Others practice it when the need arises. You can start with 10- or 20-minute sessions, and adjust the time as you see fit.

Posture
Sit in a comfortable position. Legs may be crossed if you're on the floor, a mat, or a cushion. If you're sitting in a chair, position yourself so your feet are flat on the floor if you can. Support yourself with cushions behind your back, under your knees, or elsewhere as needed. Keep your back comfortably straight, eyes closed.

Remember
Work to remain neutral about your thoughts and emotions. This isn't rumination! If you become distracted or find your mind wandering, bring your attention back to your intention. You can always turn to mindful meditation for a time if you need a break.

HOW TO DO IT

Step 1
Spend 5 to 10 minutes in mindful meditation. Focus on your breath, and let thoughts come and go.

Step 2
When you're ready, call up the event, person, period of time, or other subject you've chosen to reflect on.

Step 3
Look at the details of your subject. What images, emotions, sounds, smells, or sensations does it bring with it? If you're working through a memory of an event, what were your emotions at that time? What sights, smells, and physical sensations were you experiencing?

Step 4
Focus in turn on each image, emotion, sound, smell, or physical sensation the subject conjured in Step 3. View them as a neutral outsider might. Are there patterns? Is an aspect of the subject particularly dominant? How do the emotions and circumstances surrounding that subject compare to your current state?

Step 5
One by one, let each image, emotion, sound, smell, and physical sensation go. Take time to focus on each detail, and then let it fade from your attention as you move on to the next.

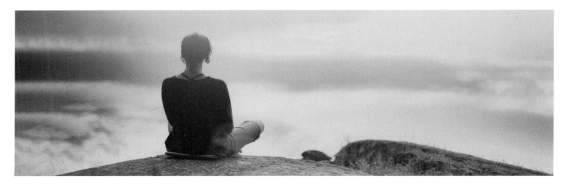

Step 6

Consider the subject as a whole for a moment, with all its aspects, and then let it fade from your attention.

Step 7

Take a few minutes to come back to simple mindfulness, focusing only on your breath.

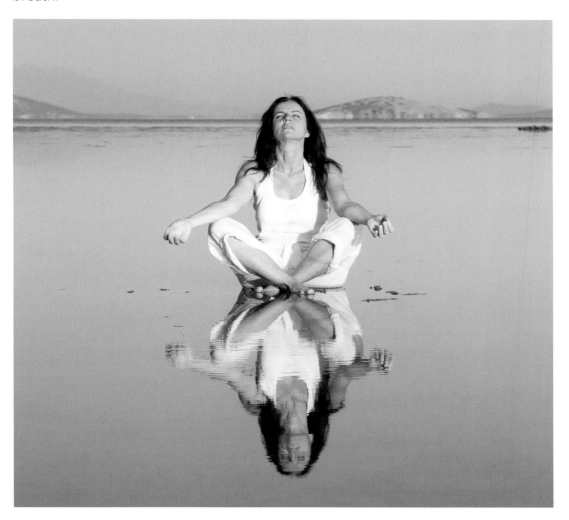

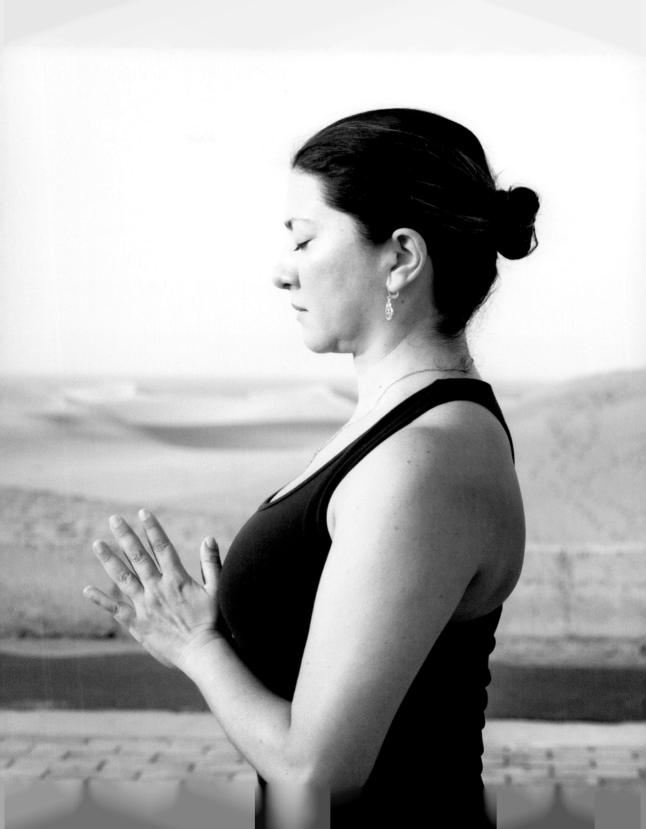

SLOW BODY MOVEMENT

You can bring laser-sharp focus to a single part of your body as you slowly move that part around. This is a kind of mindful meditation. The trick is to move slowly, so slowly that you have time to note all of the muscles, bones, and tendons that make the movement possible. You can also experience the pull of gravity, the temperature, and the movement of the air around your body in a new way. Sometimes this meditation is just about the movement. At other times, it involves a gradual stretch.

You can apply slow body movement to any part of the body. The ones described here are just a few examples to get you started.

Time
Try spending 5 or 10 minutes with this movement. You can lengthen your sessions as you become more comfortable.

Space
Make sure you have plenty of space needed to move your limbs freely.

Remember
Your mind will wander, and that's ok. When it wanders, acknowledge that it has. Then gently bring your attention back to your body.

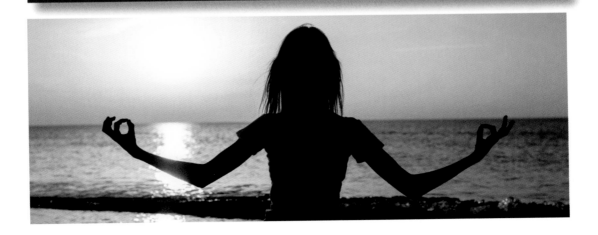

HANDS

Step 1

Come to a seated position, either on the floor with your legs crossed, or on a chair with your feet flat on the floor. Keep your back comfortably erect. You can also adjust this meditation to do it lying down.

Step 2

Rest your hands, palms down, on your knees.

Step 3

Bring your focus to your hands. What sensations are you experiencing there?

Step 4

Raise your hands very slowly and steadily until they hover at about chest height. Keep your attention on your hands and arms as they lift. Let them feel heavy as gravity pulls on them. Consider each muscle, tendon, and bone that supports this movement.

Step 5

Slowly rotate your hands so the palms face each other.

Step 6

Move the hands together until the palms touch.

Step 7

Reverse the movements. Move your hands slowly apart, rotate your palms to face down, and bring your hands down to gently rest on your knees.

ARMS

Step 1
Come to a standing position with your back comfortably erect. Let your arms hang loosely at your sides. You can also adjust this meditation to do it lying down.

Step 2
Bring your attention to your left arm, first focusing on the finger tips, then moving up to your shoulder. What sensations are you experiencing there?

Step 3
Keeping your shoulders down, lift your elbow with your hand following behind. Continue moving until your arm is pointing straight up. Focus on the feeling of this movement as you do so.

Step 4
Stretch your arm up even farther—pulling from your back, to your shoulder, up through your fingers—as though you're trying to grab an apple in a tree. You can come to your toes to reach higher.

Step 5
Reverse the movement. Come back to flat feet, if you were on your toes. Bring your arm down slowly, leading with the elbow, the hand following behind, until the arm again hangs loosely at your side.

Step 6
Repeat the movement with your right arm.

HEAD

Step 1
Come to a seated position, either on the floor with your legs crossed, or on a chair with your feet flat on the floor. Keep your back comfortably erect. You can also adjust this meditation to do it lying down.

Step 2
Bring your attention to your head and neck. If it helps, shift your head around a little. Feel the heaviness of the head as it balances on your neck.

Step 3
Keeping your shoulders still, move your head slowly forward until you're looking straight down.

Step 4
Gradually turn your head so it faces left.

Step 5
Lift your head so it sits up straight on your neck, your face looking left.

Step 6
Turn your head to face forward.

Step 7
Move your head forward until you're looking straight down, and repeat the process, this time looking to the right.

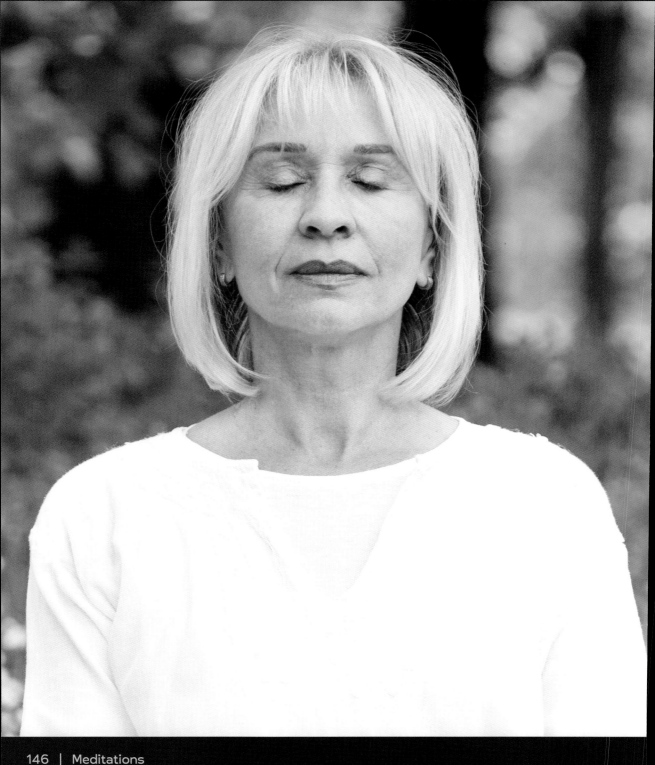

We are not going around in circles, we are moving up, the circle is a spiral, we have already ascended many a level.

—Herman Hesse

SOUND

Sound is a powerful thing. Music can inspire emotions or bring back memories. Sudden noises can annoy us, frighten us, or call us to action. Sound has been used in both medicine and entertainment. It can also play a part in meditation.

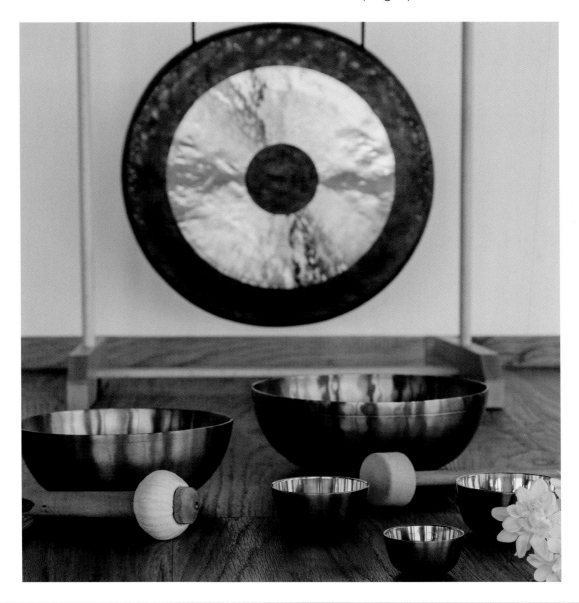

BINAURAL BEATS

When a tone entering one ear is a certain frequency, and a tone entering your other ear is a slightly different frequency, you start to hear a third tone that isn't really there. That phantom sound, or binaural beat, is pitched at the frequency between the two tones playing in your ears. For example, if one ear hears a tone at 300 Hertz and the other hears one at 305, the binaural beat's frequency is 5 Hertz. It's a phenomenon that researchers are still trying to understand, though there are many theories about what exactly it does to the brain.

There's some evidence that binaural beats affect the way your brain functions, whether by promoting deep sleep, a meditative focus, or a more accurate memory. Different frequencies are also believed to affect the brain differently.

Type	Frequency (in Hertz)	Effects
Delta	0.5–4	Helps a person enter or stay in deep, dreamless sleep
Theta	4–7	Promotes REM sleep, creative thinking, and meditation
Alpha	7–12	Helps relaxation and lessens anxiety
Beta	12–30	Improves focus, problem-solving, and memory (higher frequencies in this range can increase anxiety)
Gamma	30–50	Helps a person stay alert while awake

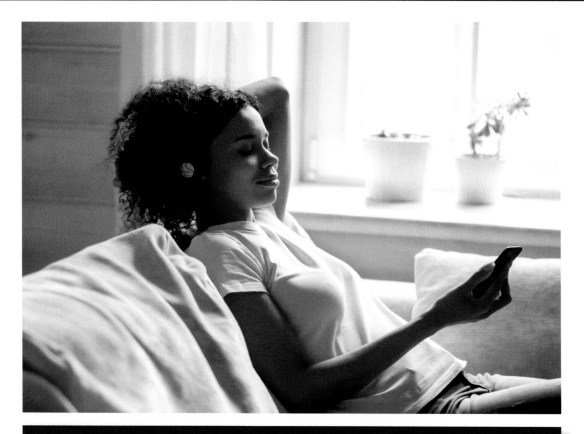

Time

It's generally agreed that the longer you spend listening to binaural beats, the more effective they are.

Posture

If meditating, assume a posture that suits the form of meditation. Otherwise, you can sit or lie comfortably, or listen as you perform other tasks, such as reading or housework.

Remember

You need headphones to listen to binaural beats. This is the only way to have different tones play in different ears. Don't listen at too loud a volume so you don't end up with damaged hearing. Avoid listening to binaural beats while trying to drive or operate heavy machinery.

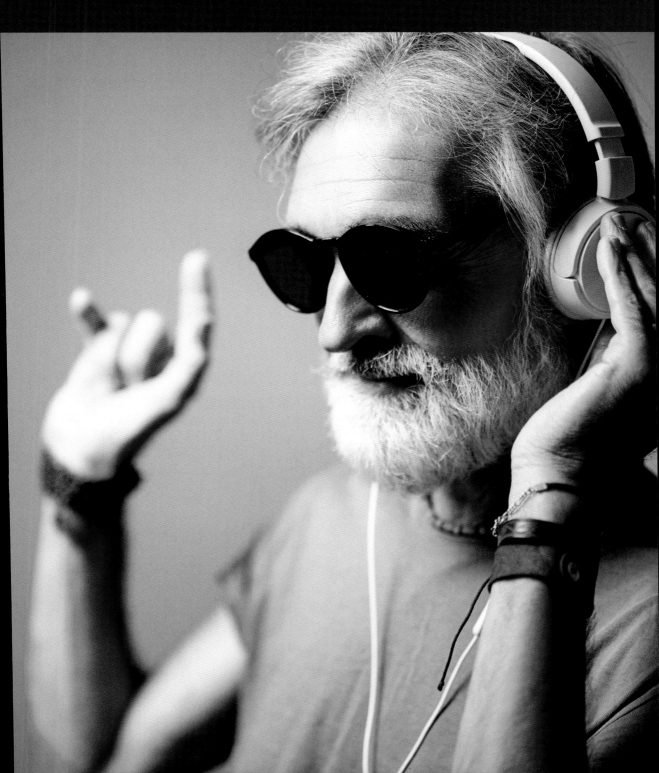

SOUND BATH

It's well known that music can help us relax. Sound baths strip the idea of calming music down to a non-melodic collection of tones, beats, or other sounds. These sounds often come from singing bowls, gongs, a shruti box (similar to a harmonium), and human vocals. They are called baths because participants often feel surrounded and submerged in the vibrations of the sounds.

Part of a sound bath's effectiveness comes from the basic, calming aspect of the sounds, which give busy minds something to do other than ruminate or plan. Many believe the physical vibrations of the sound waves, moving from the instruments, through the air, and into the body, also help bring relaxation and even healing.

You can listen to sound bath recordings, but the experience pales in comparison to a live event. Group sessions can be found at specialized businesses built around sound baths, as well as some yoga studios and spas. Some people make their own sound baths by playing a singing bowl or other instrument themselves.

Time
Depending on who is organizing the sound bath, it may last between 45 to 90 minutes. You may also be able to find ones that last longer or shorter.

Posture
Find a comfortable position. Many people lie down, with support under the knees or head as needed, with their eyes closed. Others may sit, enter a more active yoga pose, or move between positions as the mood strikes.

Remember
Let your body do what it needs to do, including fidget, change position, stretch, and yawn. Keep your mind present, however, and try not to fall asleep.

THIRD EYE

The third eye is an image that is used in many meditation discussions today. It's counted as one of the body's seven main chakras, and is located between and just above the eyes. Some people associate the third eye with enlightenment, others with empathy or intuition, and some with an understanding of the physical and spiritual worlds. Generally speaking, the third eye is believed to be "closed" when left to its own devices. With a closed third eye, you are cut off from experiencing much empathy or intuition. The goal of this meditation, then, is to open the third eye.

You can include this meditation in a practice that works through all of the seven major chakras, or focus on the third eye by itself.

Time
If you're just starting out, try meditating on the third eye for 10 to 15 minutes. You can increase that time as you become more comfortable with the practice.

Posture
Sit in a comfortable position. Legs may be crossed if you're on the floor, a mat (such as a prayer mat), or a cushion. If you're sitting in a chair, position yourself so your feet are flat on the floor if you can. Support yourself with cushions behind your back, under your knees, or elsewhere as needed. Keep your back comfortably straight, eyes closed.

Remember
Your mind will wander, and that's ok. When it wanders, acknowledge that it has. Then gently bring your attention back to the third eye.

HOW TO DO IT

Step 1
Take a few deep breaths to ground yourself. Then return to normal breathing.

Step 2
Bring your attention to the location of your third eye.

Step 3
Begin to visualize a bright ball of light energy surrounding that spot. The light glows indigo, a deep color between blue and violet.

Step 4
As you inhale and exhale, imagine the energy from your breaths making the light bigger, brighter, and warmer.

Step 5
Try to visualize a closed eye within the light.

Step 6
When the image of the closed eye becomes clear, imagine the eye opening. Hold this image in your mind.

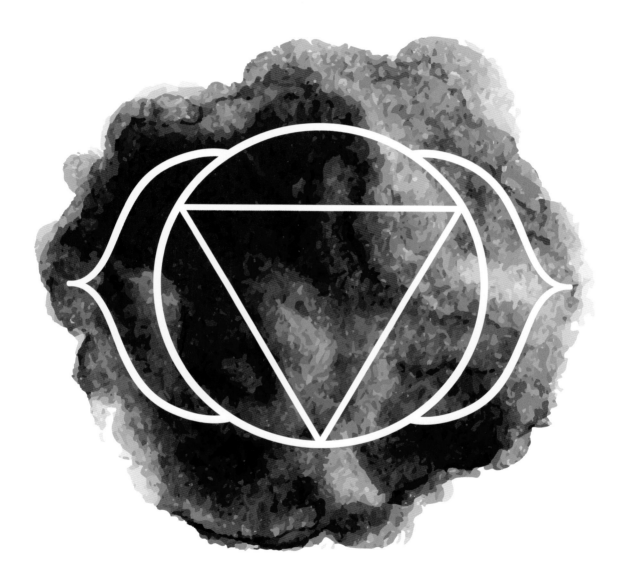

VIPASSANA

Vipassana is the oldest form of meditation in Buddhism, and over the millennia it has spread from India to the world. The word vipassana can be roughly translated as, "to see into something clearly," or "to see in a special way." Many people have used the rough English translation of "insight," which describes the driving intention of the meditation. Practicing Vipassana is meant to help you reach balance within yourself and understand the true nature of reality. You build this awareness and understanding up over the course of years.

Vipassana can be described as both gentle and thorough, as it gradually and patiently strives toward full-awareness of yourself, the world, and reality in general. The practice uses elements of mindfulness, noting, and breathing meditations to do this.

Time
As a beginner, you can start with 5 or 10 minutes. As you become more comfortable, you can extend that time. Some people practice Vipassana for hours, and meditation retreats lasting more than a week are found in many places.

Posture
Sit in a comfortable position. Legs may be crossed or in a lotus position if you're on the floor or a cushion. If you're sitting in a chair, position yourself so your feet are flat on the floor if you can. Support yourself with cushions behind your back, under your knees, or elsewhere as needed. Keep your back comfortably straight, eyes closed.

Remember
Your mind will wander, and that's ok. When it wanders, acknowledge that it has. Then gently bring your attention back to the breath.

HOW TO DO IT

Step 1
Take a few deep breaths to ground yourself. Then return to normal breathing.

Step 2
Bring your focus to the feeling of the air as it moves through your nostrils with each inhale and exhale.

Step 3
Move your attention to your abdomen, feeling the belly move out as you inhale, and in as you exhale. If it helps, repeat "rising" in your mind as you inhale, and "falling" as you exhale.

Step 4
Note any sounds, smells, tastes, or physical sensations you experience. Label your experience of them ("hearing," "smelling," "tasting," "touching") and let them go.

Step 5
As thoughts and emotions come up, note that you are "thinking," "feeling," then let them go.

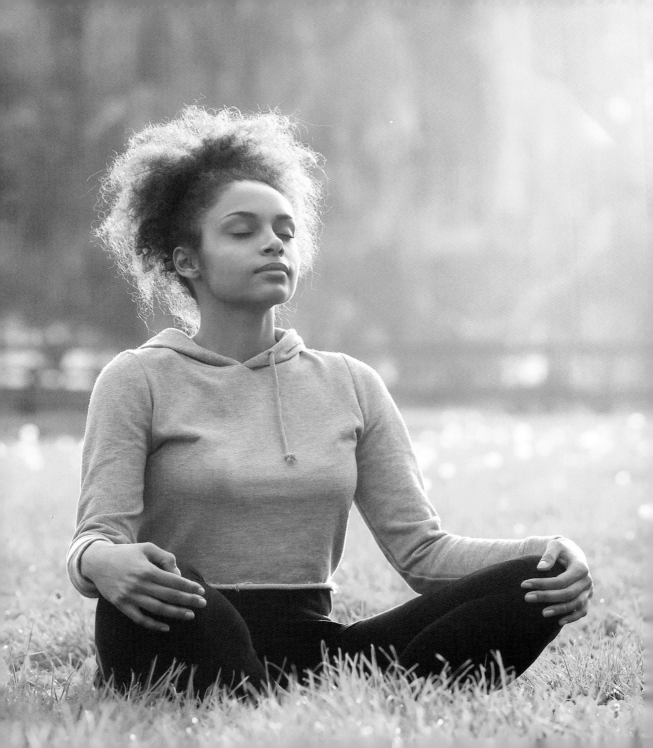

This mind of mine went formerly wandering about as it liked, as it listed, as it pleased; but I shall now hold it in thoroughly, as the rider who holds the hook holds in the furious elephant.

—the Dhammapada

WALKING MEDITATION

Not all meditation is about sitting still. Walking meditation involves bringing deliberate mindfulness to each step you take. Like other mindfulness exercises, walking meditation can help you cultivate a clearer mind and reduce some of your stress.

Time
If you're practicing this meditation for the first time, you can keep a session relatively short. Try a five-minute session. See how you feel and adjust from there. Experienced practitioners may meditate for 45 minutes or more.

Posture
Keep your back comfortably straight. Your neck should be long, and your gaze relaxed and down. Your hands can hang loosely at your sides, or you can gently clasp your hands in front or behind you.

Pace
You'll walk much more slowly as you meditate than you do when you're just walking to a destination. Walk slow enough that you can give each stage of each step the attention it deserves. Keep a steady, even rhythm.

Remember
Your mind will wander, and that's okay. If you have trouble bringing it back to a meditative focus, there are a couple of things to try:

- Pause in your walking and address the distraction. Why is it demanding your attention? Is it a tumultuous thought, a beautiful sight, or a loud sound? Stop for as long as you need. When you're able to bring your attention back to walking, continue on.

- It may help to increase or decrease your pace slightly.

HOW TO DO IT

Step 1
Find a spot inside or outside where you can walk 10 to 15 paces safely and with few distractions.

Step 2
Take your first step:
Raise the heel of one foot.
Lift the foot off the ground.
Move the foot forward, feeling your body shift its weight as it does so.
Drop the foot gently to the ground, heel first.
Press the sole of the foot into the ground.

Step 3
Repeat the process with the other foot. Continue step-by-step, focusing on each sensation as it arises, each muscle as it flexes and relaxes.

Step 4
When you've gone 10 to 15 steps, turn around and return to your starting spot. Then turn and start again.

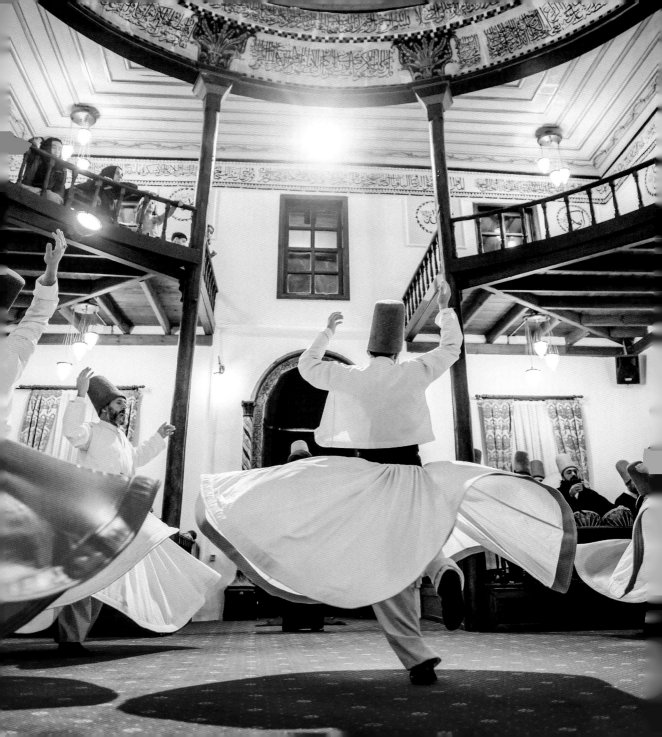

WHIRLING

Sema, often called whirling in English, is a meditative dance practiced in the Mevlevi order of Sufism. The meditation practice is centered on the act of spinning, as music plays in the background. Formal practitioners receive a huge amount of training—perhaps 1,000 days—before becoming fully involved in the Sema ceremony as dervishes. When practicing Sema, trained dervishes can spin continuously for as long as an hour, without ever feeling dizzy.

As they practice, dervishes strive toward ecstasy and a direct connection to God, as well as ridding themselves of their individual egos. Their clothing reflects this last point: the tall, conical hat represents the ego's tombstone, and the long white robe is the ego's death shroud.

Time
Whirling takes practice. Try starting with perhaps 30 seconds of spinning, then resting, and work up from there. Take your time extending the length of your practice—remember that trained dervishes receive years of training.

Space
Make sure you have the space needed to move freely. The floor should be clear of obstacles.

Remember
Your mind will wander, and that's ok. When it wanders, acknowledge that it has. Then gently bring your attention back to your movement.

HOW TO DO IT

Step 1
Cross your arms in front of you, right over left, so each hand rests on the opposite shoulder. Bow to the space where you'll be whirling, and to the divine.

Step 2
Begin to whirl slowly, counterclockwise, pivoting on your right foot. Your gaze should be relaxed and unfocused.

Step 3
Start to unfurl your arms from their crossed positions, raising them gradually until they arch up.

Step 4
Speed up gradually.

Step 5
When you're ready to end the practice, slow your spin gradually. Stand a moment, then kneel and touch your forehead to the floor.

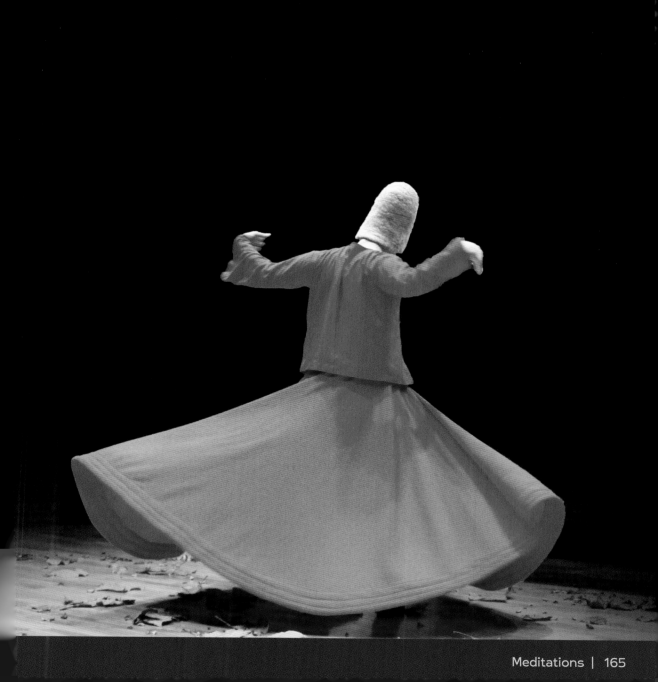

Be silent that the Lord who gave thee language may speak,

For as He fashioned a door and lock, He has also made a key.

—Rumi

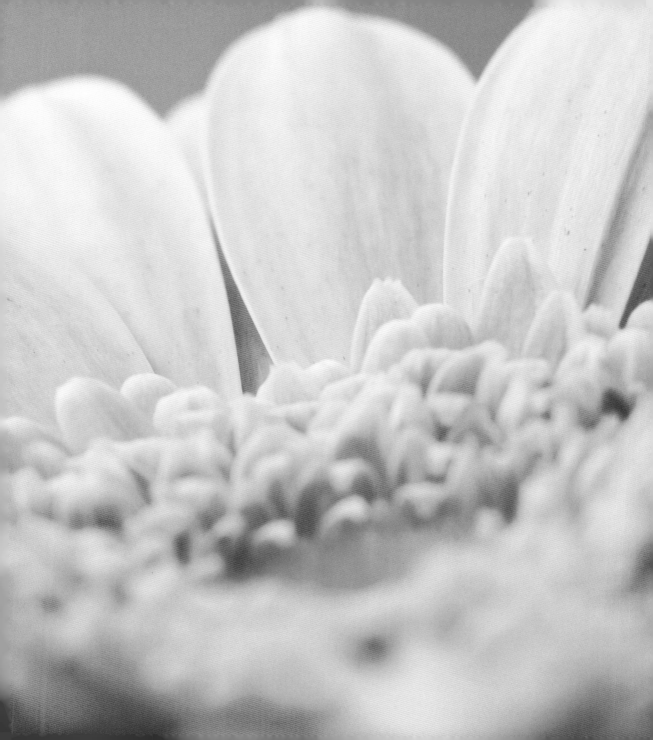

YOGA

What we often think of as yoga today is an adaptation of a Hindu practice first written about millennia ago. Classical yoga is defined by disciplined physical, mental, and spiritual exercises. These are practiced to help achieve oneness with the divine or supreme knowledge.

Today, yoga encompasses a range of paths to follow, each of which focuses on different techniques. There are yogas that use sounds or images. Some paths make more use of breath control, while others prioritize mental concentration. There are also the practices that focus most on physical exercises.

People also come to yoga with a variety of goals. Nowadays, not all yogis are working toward union with the divine. Some people come for relaxation, others for improvements to their strength, flexibility, or mental discipline. If you explore yoga, ask yourself what your intentions are with the practice. Some paths will serve those intentions better than others. Of course, you can also switch from one practice to another, or combine them for the best fit.

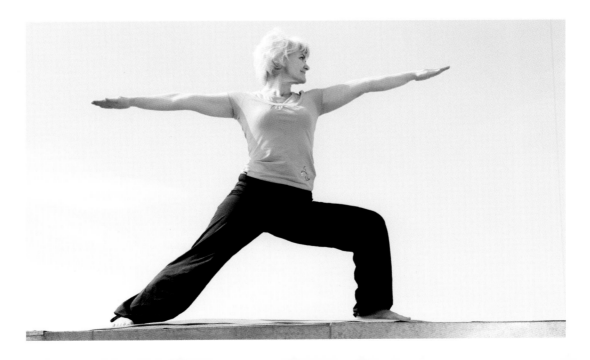

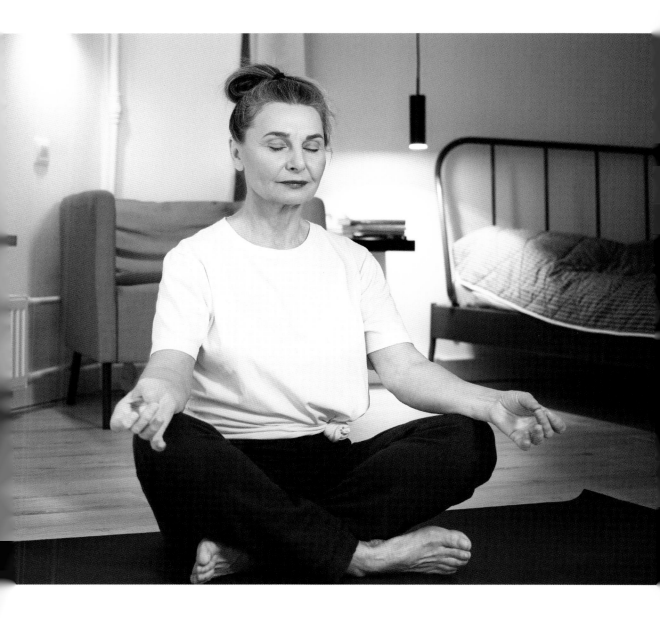

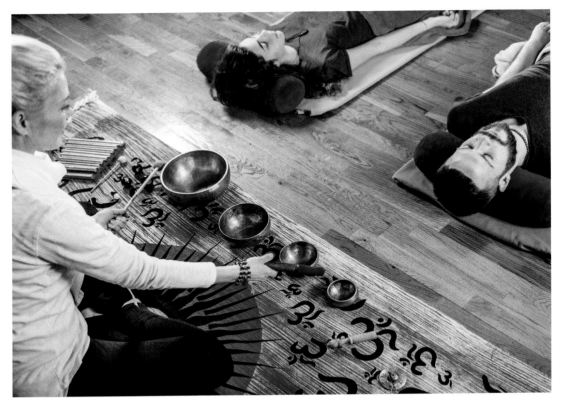

NADA YOGA

Nada can be translated as "sound" in Sanskrit. This yoga of sound is based on the idea that a person can use sound to access a higher state of being.

Sound can be divided roughly into four types:
1. Coarse vocal sound: Sounds you hear with your ears, such as music, speech, or footsteps.
2. Finer vocal sound: Quieter sounds that require concentration to hear, such as whispering.
3. Mental or visualized sound: Sounds heard only in your mind, often accompanied by shapes or colors.
4. Para, or transcendental sound: a sound at such a high frequency that it is well beyond hearing and perhaps beyond vibration; it is, in effect, the "universal consciousness" experienced as sound.

Time
You can spend 10 to 15 minutes with Nada yoga as a beginner. As you become more comfortable with the practice, you can meditate for longer.

Posture
Sit in a comfortable position. Legs may be crossed if you're on the floor. You can also sit on a sturdy pillow or rolled-up blanket in a squat position, with your legs straddling the support and your feet flat on the floor. If you're sitting in a chair, position yourself so your feet are flat on the floor if you can. Support yourself with cushions behind your back, under your knees, or elsewhere as needed. Keep your back comfortably straight, gaze lowered or eyes closed. Rest your hands on your knees, or press your thumbs gently into your ears and support your forehead with your fingers, resting your elbows on your knees or a table.

Remember
Your mind will wander, and that's ok. When it wanders, acknowledge that it has. Then gently bring your attention back to the sound.

HOW TO DO IT

Step 1

Choose a mantra. A short, 1- or 2-syllable sound might be a good one to start with. Repeat it steadily and strongly aloud. Listen to the vibration of it.

Step 2

Change your chanting to a whisper, or just mouth the mantra. Stay connected to the sound of the mantra.

Step 3

When you're ready, stop chanting aloud and repeat the mantra in your mind. Acknowledge any images, shapes, or colors that appear.

Step 4

Your awareness of any other sound should start to drop away.
As it does, let your conscious chanting of the mantra fade.
Listen to the sound—or silence—it leaves behind.

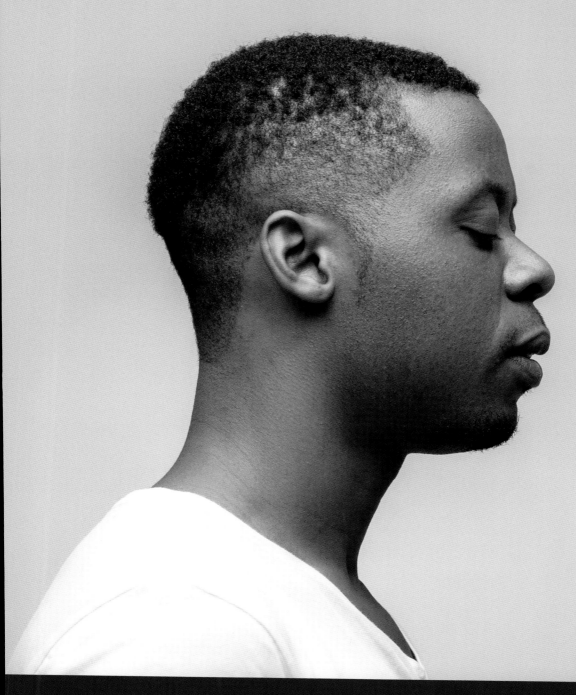

KUNDALINI YOGA

Kundalini yoga is a practice that combines body postures, mantras, breath control, and mental focus. The word roughly means "coiled," and it refers to an energy that is believed to be trapped at the base of everyone's spine. The point of practicing kundalini is to "uncoil" this energy, awakening it and directing it through the body. This provides awareness of and connection to the higher self.

Time
Classes usually last an hour or an hour and a half.

Clothing and Supplies
Clothing should be comfortable and made from natural fibers such as cotton or linen. Yogis often wear turbans or other head coverings made of the same material. Your mat should either be made of natural fibers or covered in a blanket made of natural fibers.

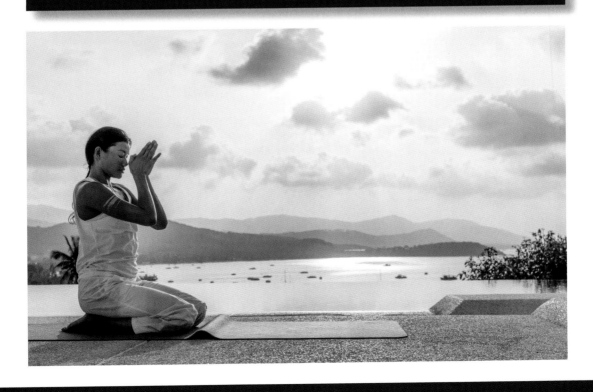

CONTENT OF A SESSION

Chant
Many people start a session with kundalini off by repeating "Ong Namo Guru Dev Namo" a few times. This is a respectful acknowledgement to the creative energy and divine teacher within each of us.

Warm Up
A few minutes are spent doing some simple movements to prepare the body, particularly the spine, for movement.

Movement
About half of the session is taken up by a kriya, which is a series of body postures, "locks" or bandhas (muscle contractions), and breathing techniques.

Relaxation
Movement is followed by a few minutes in quiet contemplation. Practitioners generally lie in shavasana pose, on the back with arms and legs extended.

Seated Meditation
A session ends with a seated meditation. In a group setting, this often involves mantras, though not always.

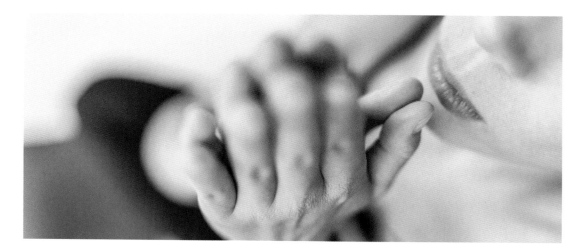

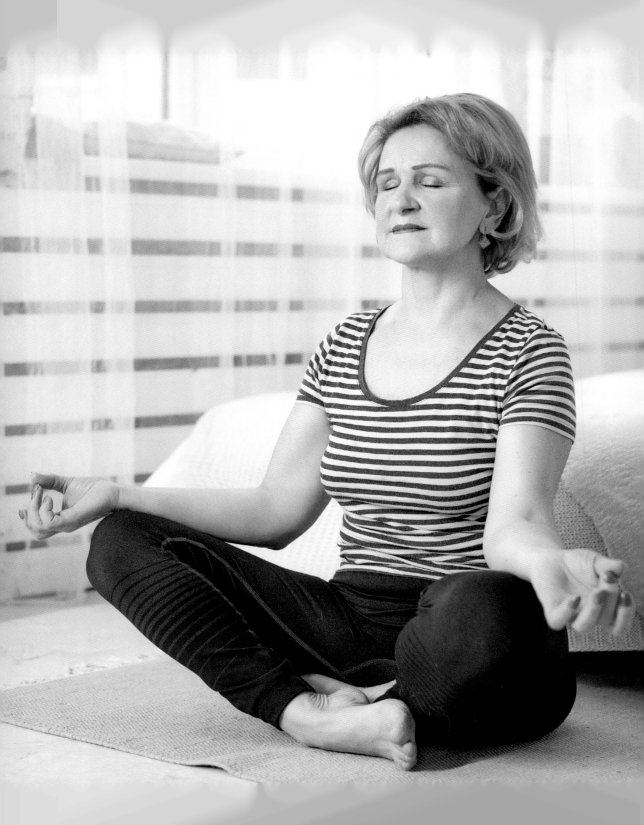

HATHA YOGA

Hatha yoga is a category that includes what you see in most yoga studios in the United States. This is the yoga of physical movement and poses. Vinyasa, Bikram, and Ashtanga yoga all fit under this umbrella. (That said, studios often use "Hatha yoga" to refer specifically to classes that spend long stretches of time in each pose.)

Time
It's a good idea to spend at least 15 minutes doing a sequence of yoga poses. Many people spend an hour or more. Each pose may be held for anywhere from a few breaths to several minutes. Moving between a lot of different poses in quick succession requires more stamina. Slower-paced sequences that spend several minutes in each pose tend to be more relaxing.

Supplies
Clothing should be comfortable and made from natural fibers such as cotton or linen. Yogis often wear turbans or other head coverings made of the same material. Your mat should either be made of natural fibers or covered in a blanket made of natural fibers.

Remember
Yoga should challenge you, but it should never cause pain or injury. Listen to your body throughout your practice, and adjust poses or take a rest when you need to.

There are a lot of different poses. The next pages describe a few basic ones.

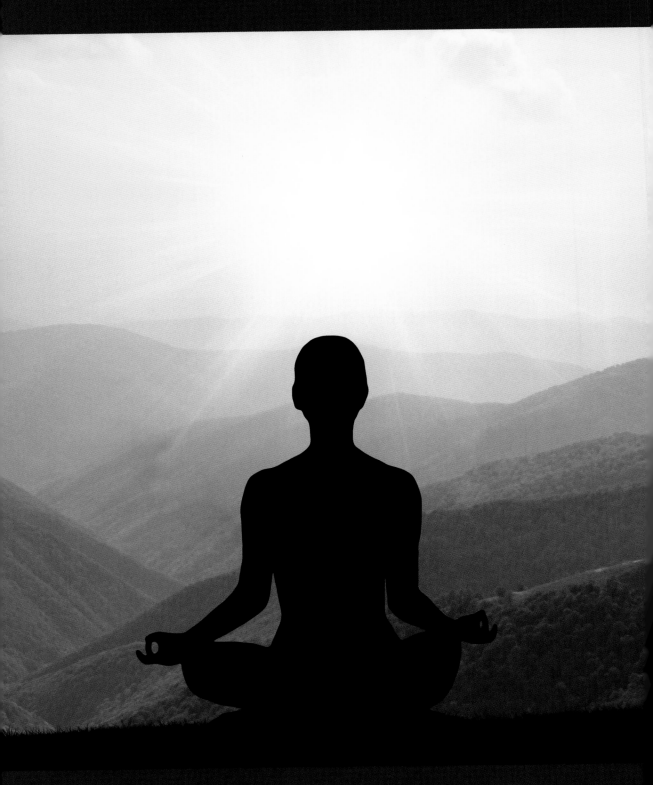

Child's Pose

1. Start on hands and knees, in a tabletop position. Your hands should be directly below your shoulders, and your knees should be directly below your hips.

2. Move your knees apart. Aim for perhaps 12 inches between your knees. They can be wider or closer together depending on what is comfortable to you. Your big toes should touch.

3. Move your hips back and down. Let them rest on or near your heels.

4. Rest your belly on your thighs and your forehead on the mat.

5. Extend your arms to the front with palms down. You can also lay your arms along your sides, fingers pointing behind you.

6. Breathe deeply.

Modify:

If you experience any pain or discomfort, you can place a pillow, blanket, or other support under your hips, knees, head, or torso. This lessens the stretch and helps you avoid straining any joints.

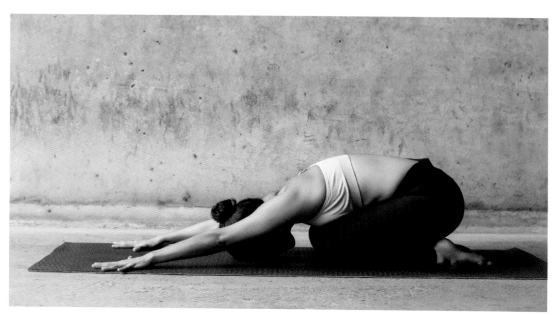

Cat and Cow Pose Sequence

1. Start on hands and knees, in a tabletop position.

2. Inhale and your arch your back, from hip to head, making a U shape (a bit like a cow's back). Lengthen your neck away from the shoulders and look out ahead of you or slightly up.

3. Exhale, rounding your back up (like an angry cat). Draw your belly in and look at your bellybutton.

4. Repeat. Move between an arched and a rounded back in a smooth cycle.

Modify:

Though two separate poses, cat and cow are generally done together in a sequence that is repeated over several breaths.

Reclined Spinal Twist

1. Lie on your back, knees bent and feet flat on the floor.

2. Move both knees together to your right, resting them stacked on the floor if possible.

3. Extend your left arm out to your left, and move your head to look to the left.

4. Repeat on the other side.

Modify:

If your shoulders and neck are tight, you can try putting a blanket or pillow under your head for support.

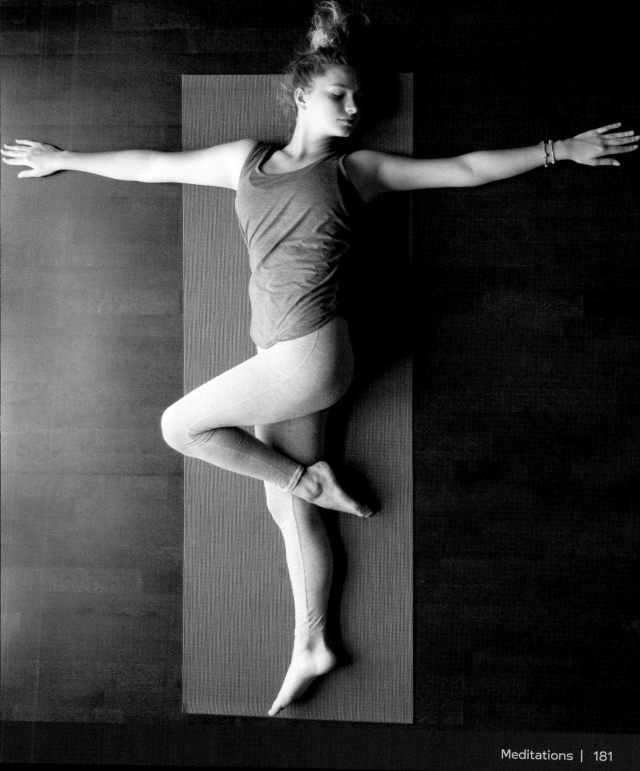

Forward Fold

1. Stand tall, feet placed hip-width apart and knees in a slight bend.

2. Bend forward, hinging from the hips and keeping your back long.

3. Extend your arms toward the ground or grab opposite elbows.

Modify:

You can also do this pose with your legs in a wide V.

Downward-Facing Dog

1. Start in a push-up position, with hands directly under shoulders and body long. Your knees can be lifted or resting on the ground.
2. Point fingers and toes forward. Stretch your fingers apart.
3. Lift your hips up and back, knees off the floor, into an upside-down V shape.
4. Extend your back to be as long as possible, with strong, straight arms.

Modify:

Your legs don't have to be perfectly straight or your heels flat on the floor. Work toward these positions gradually.

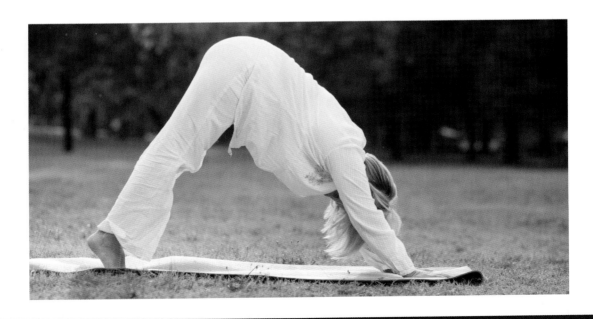

Corpse Pose

1. Lie flat on your back.

2. Extend your legs out and relax them. Your feet will naturally turn out a little.

3. Extend your arms along your sides, palms up.

4. Close your eyes.

Modify:

Keep knees bent and feet flat on the floor if your lower back is uncomfortable. You may also use a pillow, blanket, or other support to lift your head, knees, or calves.

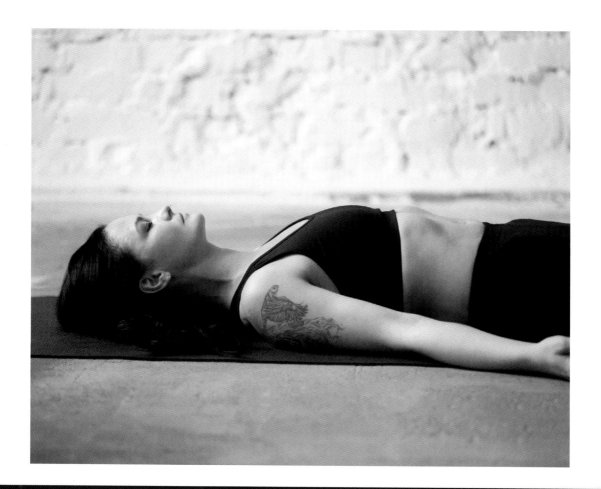

Like any other science, yoga is applicable to people of every clime and time. Yoga is a method for restraining the natural turbulence of thoughts, which otherwise impartially prevent all men, of all lands, from glimpsing their true nature. Yoga cannot know a barrier of East and West any more than does the healing and equitable light of the sun. So long as man possesses a mind with its restless thoughts, so long will there be a universal need for yoga.

—Paramahansa Yogananda

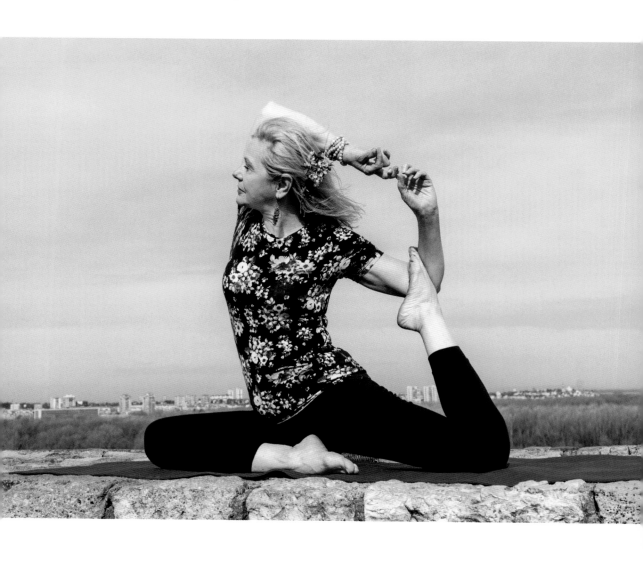

ZAZEN

Zazen is practiced in the Zen school of Buddhism. A core Zen belief is that anyone can achieve awakening, or enlightenment. The school also emphasizes a one-ness among all living and non-living things. Both of these concepts shape zazen. It's a very intentional form of meditation that involves getting rid of individual identity—including likes or dislikes, desires, expectations, and goals—to exist in the present moment, as well as becoming aware of the breath, body, and mind as a single, complete unit.

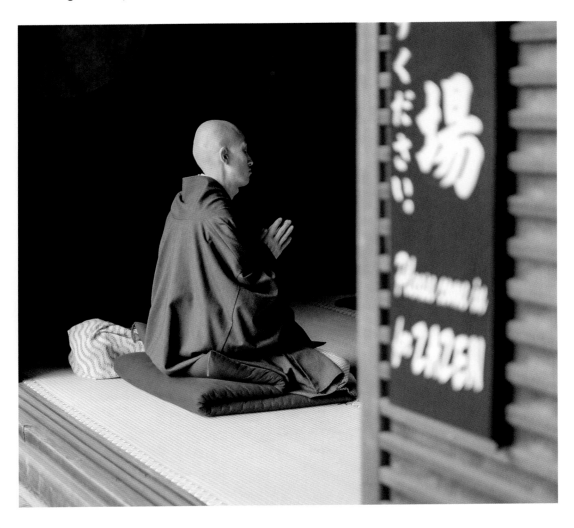

Time
Devotees often practice zazen for 20 to 30 minutes, one or two times a day. If you're a beginner, you can work up to this kind of practice gradually.

Posture
The body's position is an important part of zazen practice.

Legs: You have a few options. In all poses, you can sit on a support to make the position easier to do.
- Full lotus: Sit cross-legged with each foot resting on top of the opposite thigh.
- Half lotus: One foot rests on the opposite thigh, the other foot is folded underneath the opposite leg.
- Seiza: Kneel, resting your hips on your heels. You can sit on a cushion (legs on either side) or low bench (legs folded under the bench) to make this position more comfortable.
- Chair: Sit near the edge of the chair so your back is straight and your feet rest flat on the floor. Place a cushion between your lower back and the chair back if you need some support.

Hands: Lay your hands together on your lap, palms up. Rest the fingers of one hand on top of the other, with your dominant hand on bottom (if you're right-handed, your right hand is on bottom, and vice versa for left-handers). Let the tips of your thumbs touch so your hands form an oval shape.

Spine: Keep your back comfortably erect. Tuck your chin slightly to lengthen your neck.

Eyes: Allow your gaze to rest, eyes open and unfocused, a few feet in front of you.

Remember
Your mind will wander, and that's ok. When it wanders, acknowledge that it has. Then gently bring your attention back to the breath.

HOW TO DO IT

Step 1
Take a moment to settle into your seated position.

Step 2
Bring your attention to your breath.
- Your breathing should be easy and comfortable, not controlled.
- Breathe through your nose, your mouth closed and relaxed.
- Rest your tongue gently against the roof of your mouth, just behind your front teeth.

Step 3
Counting your inhales and exhales in the beginning can help you calm and focus your mind. As your mind quietens, let the counting go and just breathe. If it helps to label your thoughts and sensations in the beginning, do so, but let this go with time, too.

Step 4
Move your focus to the physical sensation of breathing, whether it's your belly moving in and out, or the air entering and leaving your lungs. If there are changes in the speed or rhythm of your breathing, note them.

Step 5
Work toward experiencing your breath as a continuous cycle. Forget any notion of parts or stages of the breath, such as inhale, pause, or exhale. It is a single, unbroken movement.

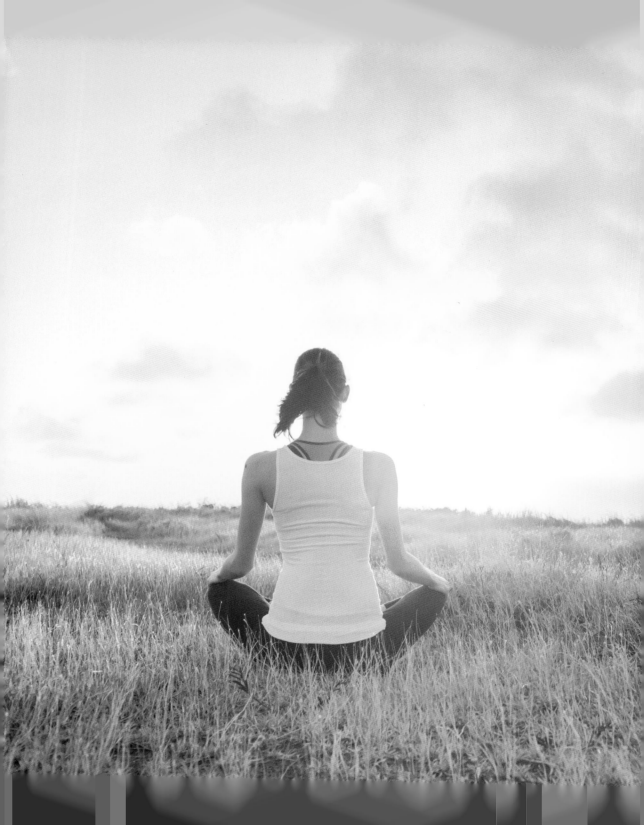

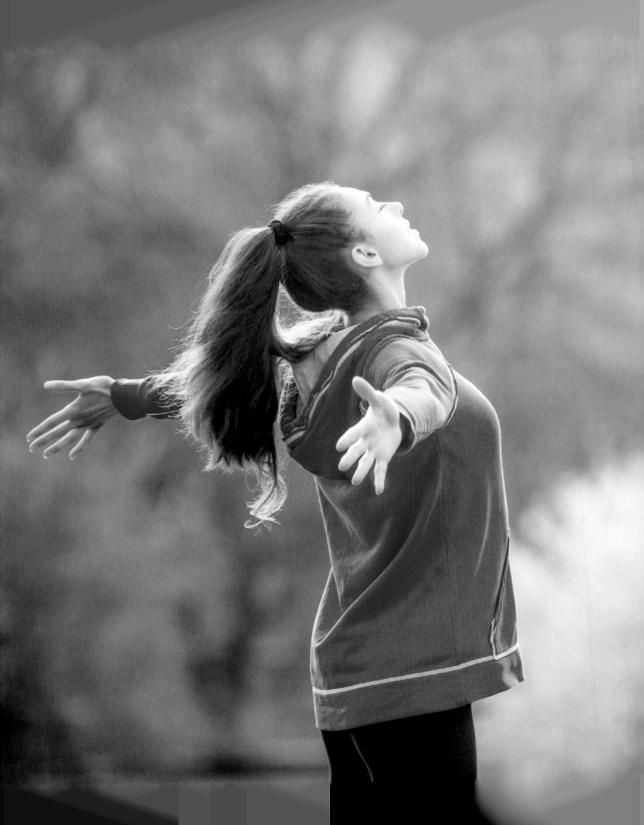